Research Report

Developing Navy Capability to Recover Forces in Chemical, Biological, and Radiological Hazard Environments

Adam C. Resnick, Steven A. Knapp

Prepared for the Office of the Secretary of Defense
Approved for public release; distribution unlimited

RAND NATIONAL DEFENSE RESEARCH INSTITUTE

The research described in this report was sponsored by OPNAV N81 and conducted within the Forces and Resources Policy Center of the RAND National Defense Research Institute, a federally funded research and development center sponsored by OSD, the Joint Staff, the Unified Combatant Commands, the Navy, the Marine Corps, the defense agencies, and the defense Intelligence Community.

Library of Congress Cataloging-in-Publication Data

Resnick, Adam C.
Developing Navy capability to recover forces in chemical, biological, and radiological hazard environments / Adam C. Resnick, Steven A. Knapp.
pages cm
Includes bibliographical references.
ISBN 978-0-8330-8147-6 (pbk. : alk. paper)
1. Amphibious warfare—Planning. 2. United States. Navy—Planning. 3. United States. Navy—Operational readiness. 4. Decontamination (from gases, chemicals, etc.) 5. Biological decontamination. 6. Radioactive decontamination. I. Knapp, Steven A. II. Title.e.
U261.R47 2013
359.9'646—dc23

2013037115

RAND OFFICES

SANTA MONICA, CA • WASHINGTON, DC

PITTSBURGH, PA • NEW ORLEANS, LA • JACKSON, MS • BOSTON, MA

DOHA, QA • CAMBRIDGE, UK • BRUSSELS, BE

www.rand.org

Preface

In 2010, the Director of the Assessments Division in the office of the Chief of Naval Operations (OPNAV N81) expressed concern that the Navy lacked clearly defined capabilities to recover contaminated forces during amphibious operations.

The mission to recover amphibious forces ashore will present challenges if forces come under attack from chemical, biological, or radiological (CBR) weapons. If attacked with CBR weapons, contaminated forces will pose a risk of cross-contaminate to other forces during recovery and decontamination processes. Additionally, contamination will likely spread to equipment and vehicles, creating persistent hazards.

The Navy sought policy options to increase its capability to recover ashore forces while maximizing remaining battle group capability. Policy options should address conditions under which forces are recovered after being thoroughly decontaminated ashore and when they are recovered prior. Guidance should be provided to support selection of connector to recover, and ship to receive forces. Methods should be defined and developed to decontaminate forces and mitigate cross-contamination both while forces are en route and when they arrive at the sea base. Current capacity to recover forces and prospects to return the battle group to full mission capability should be identified.

The research approach included gathering data through literature review and interviews with subject matter experts. The analysis was refined to include only connectors and ships well-suited to recovering contaminated forces in amphibious missions. The analysis focused on the mission to transport, recover, and decontaminate forces. Medical treatment of casualties en route and the effect of CBR injuries on the demand for medical care at the sea base or after evacuation out of theater were not addressed. An FOUO version of this report (RR-155/1-OSD), available from RAND, includes several additional passages describing Navy capability to receive patients and isolate contaminated service members at sea.

The authors would like to thank their sponsor, Captain Robert Mitton, then head of the Medical Analysis Branch of the Assessments Division in the office of the Chief of Naval Operations, for his project guidance, and their action officers, Commander Brian Tolbert and Commander Eric Timmens. We also thank the representatives from DoD services, offices, and agencies who shared their expertise on all aspects of hazard response and amphibious operations, and provided us with access to data that enabled this project to be a success. Thank you to Dr. Robert Kadlec and to RAND colleague Paul DeLuca for their very thoughtful and thorough reviews of the manuscript. Finally, at RAND, we wish to thank John Winkler, National Security Research Division Forces and Resources Policy Center Director, and Jennifer Lewis, Associate Director, for their insightful comments and assistance.

This research was sponsored by OPNAV N81 and conducted within the Forces and Resources Policy Center of the RAND National Defense Research Institute, a federally funded research and development center sponsored by the Office of the Secretary of Defense, the Joint Staff, the Unified Combatant Commands, the Navy, the Marine Corps, the defense agencies, and the defense Intelligence Community.

For more information on the RAND Forces and Resources Policy Center, see http://www.rand.org/nsrd/ndri/centers/frp.html or contact the director (contact information is provided on the web page).

Contents

Figures

Tables

Summary

The mission to recover amphibious forces can be complicated if ashore forces come under attack from enemy weapons, particularly chemical, biological, or radiological (CBR) weapons. If ashore forces are attacked with CBR weapons, they may become contaminated and pose a cross-contamination risk to other forces with whom they come in contact. If contaminants spread to equipment and vehicles, creating persistent hazards, these items may pose an additional cross-contamination risk. Among the potential agents that may be used in CBR weapons, persistent liquid and solid chemical agents present the greatest challenge for physical decontamination.

Navy military capability will be compromised as ships' resources are dedicated to recover contaminated ashore forces. The personnel dedicated to the recovery mission will be directed away from their other responsibilities. Areas of ships used in the recovery mission will be unusable for other activities during the recovery process, and for the duration until they are determined to be free of any potential contaminants. Navy capability will be further degraded as personnel who are injured by CBR agents become casualties, and as conventional casualties become contaminated with CBR agents that exacerbate their underlying medical conditions.

In 2010, a series of tabletop exercises[1] conducted by the Navy revealed specific issues in Navy doctrine and capabilities related to transporting contaminated forces from land to the sea base and decontaminating contaminated forces aboard ships. Although the preference is to decontaminate ashore forces in the operating environment or in a clean area elsewhere on land, this is not always feasible. Thus, it is necessary for the Navy to have effective capabilities to recover and decontaminate affected forces aboard ships. Participants in the exercise expressed concern that the Navy lacked clearly defined capabilities to recover contaminated forces. Issues of concern included the following:

1. Which amphibious assault ship should receive contaminated forces?
2. Which connector is best to go ashore and bring forces back to the sea base?
3. What procedures should be used to decontaminate the forces when they arrive aboard the ships?
4. What is the prognosis for connectors and ships returning to full military capability in support of the mission?
5. Will the ships be required to return to port for reconstitution?

To address the capabilities identified in these exercises, researchers from RAND National Defense Research Institute (NDRI) were contracted by OPNAV N81 to assess current policies and capabilities pertaining to the recovery and decontamination of ashore forces and to identify

[1] Naval Surface Warfare Center Dahlgren Division (NSWCDD), Navy Craft CBRN Survivability TTX Status Report May 2010.

policy options the Navy could pursue to better perform this mission. RAND designed a study addressing the Navy capabilities required to perform the following amphibious mission functions:

- Transport contaminated and injured forces from shore to ship
- Decontaminate and treat litter-bound casualties at the sea base
- Decontaminate ambulatory and uninjured forces
- Return ships and transports to full mission capability.

Current Navy processes and measures of capability were documented on the basis of current military guidance and interviews with service members. Some aspects of Navy capability, such as the time necessary to transport contaminated forces from shore to ship using each of the connectors in the study, were calculated using basic spreadsheet models populated with numerical data derived from current guidance, Navy damage control crew interviews, and basic assumptions. No operational tests of capability were performed in this study.

The ashore force used in this analysis was a Marine Expeditionary Unit, which consists of approximately 3,000 Marines—all of whom were assumed to be ashore during the mission. Of this group, the study assumed that 10 percent of the force was contaminated during operations, requiring recovery to a sea base for decontamination.[2] In addition, 100 of those contaminated were also wounded in action with conventional injuries. The recovery operation involved 300 total contaminated service members, including 24 contaminated litter casualties and 75 contaminated ambulatory casualties. This is a robust but realistic scenario against which to measure the Navy's capabilities.

The study design considered alternatives for both the receiving ship and transport vehicles. It evaluated recovery to an amphibious assault group composed of Landing Helicopter Dock (LHD), Landing Platform Dock (LPD), and Landing Ship Dock (LSD) ships. Connectors analyzed for the recovery mission to transport forces from land to the sea base included the CH-46 Sea Knight, CH-53E Sea Stallion, MV-22 Osprey, Landing Craft Air Cushion (LCAC), and Landing Craft Utility (LCU).

The study began with an assessment of current Navy decontamination processes and capabilities. Then, using the assumptions outlined above, it evaluated steps that could be taken to increase capabilities.

Methods to Increase Navy Capability

The assessment of current Navy capability was structured around four amphibious mission functions—transporting forces, receiving casualties, decontaminating forces, and returning ships to full mission capability. After evaluating existing capabilities it was determined that the Navy

[2] U.S. Army Medical Department Center and School (USAMEDDC&S), *Multiservice Tactics, Techniques, and Procedures for Health Service Support in a Chemical, Biological, Radiological, and Nuclear Environment*, FM4-02.7/MCRP 4-11.1F/NTTP 4-02.7/AFTTP 3-42.3, July 2009.

could develop procedures to increase its throughput to recover contaminated forces by staging expedient decontamination stations and showers.

In addition, it appears that the Navy lacks a decision process for responding to a recovery mission involving CBR contamination. Once it is known that forces must be recovered, the operational commander must immediately determine what amphibious assault ship should receive contaminated forces, what connector should be used to transport forces, what procedures are required to decontaminate the forces when they arrive aboard their ship, and what decontamination processes are needed for the connectors and ships themselves.

Which amphibious assault ship should receive contaminated forces?

To minimize the opportunity cost to the battle group, forces should be recovered to one amphibious assault ship if possible. Of the amphibious assault ships in this study, the LHD has the most medical department resources[3] and should be considered to receive contaminated forces when necessary.

Which connector is best to go ashore and bring forces back to the sea base?

The selection of a connector depends on the number of forces to be recovered and how many require medical care. In cases where casualties require urgent medical attention, it is recommended that aircraft be used to recover forces—because the difference in transport time could well affect the lives of those injured. When the number of contaminated forces exceeds the passenger capacity of a single craft performing a single sortie, it is recommended that the next-largest connector be used. This policy will generally enable all forces to leave the shore as quickly as possible in a single sortie, and will minimize contamination to craft. However, operational factors may support using multiple sorties. In cases where casualties require urgent medical care and the number of forces to recover exceeds aircraft capacity, an aircraft is recommended to recover casualties and a landing craft to recover the balance of forces.

What procedures should be used to decontaminate the forces when they arrive aboard the ships?

Developing capability to increase throughput to decontaminate forces represents the greatest opportunity for the Navy to increase its capability to recover contaminated forces. *RAND recommends that the Navy increase its ability to decontaminate litter patients by staging expedient deck decontamination stations and expedient decontamination showers*. Doing so increases the throughput rate for patient decontamination and keeps contaminants toward the downwind aft section of amphibious assault ships, expediting the process to decontaminate ships and return them to full military capability. This process also keeps liquid and vapor hazards away from the fore sections of the ship, so that a vapor hazard buffer may be established and flight

---

[3] Department of the Navy, *Contingency Fact Book*, Washington D.C., Bureau of Medicine and Surgery, 2006a.

crews and other ship's crew may operate without Joint Service Lightweight Integrated Suit Technology (JSLIST) gear.

Patient Decontamination Station

Staff on amphibious assault ships should construct expedient deck patient decontamination stations. Using tables and tarps, ships' crew members can construct a three-stage process in which litter bearers or other crew members cut patients out of their protective gear and decontaminate patients while medical department representatives inspect patients to ensure that they are decontaminated.

If conditions permit, staging these expedient deck patient decontamination stations on the aft of the flight deck, in close proximity to where casualties have been recovered by aircraft, is preferred. On the aft section of the flight deck, liquid hazards carried with contaminated forces will remain on the surface of the flight deck and can easily be washed with the ship's Countermeasures Washdown System (CMWDS) after patients have been decontaminated and the aft flight deck is cleared.

Keeping contaminants aft of the superstructure on LHDs will allow continued operations on the fore sections of the ship, including flight operations. As such, flight operations can continue without requiring service members to wear protective gear. Additionally, if no hazards are detected, crew may enter and exit the interior of the ship without using decontamination stations.

Ambulatory and Uninjured Personnel Decontamination

Damage control staff are currently trained to perform personnel decontamination by setting up a contamination control area in close proximity to where forces enter the ship. After removing recovered forces' outer gear and outer garments, damage control crew escort them along a marked path toward the existing personnel decontamination stations and use the stations to process the contaminated forces. By establishing expedient showers near the area where forces board an amphibious assault ship, the Navy can gain capability by keeping liquid and vapor contaminants from permeating throughout the ship, and can perform personnel decontamination much more quickly.

In the case where ambulatory and uninjured forces arrive on the aft section of the flight deck, fire hoses outfitted with fog nozzles that reduce pressure to around 60 pounds per square inch can be used as showers.[4] Showers should be directed so that contaminated runoff drains off the ship. After showering, service members can walk upwind toward the fore section of the flight deck and the superstructure, into an area free of hazards. With this procedure, all liquid and vapor hazards remain on the aft section of the flight deck and do not interrupt operations in other areas of the ship.

---

[4] U.S. Army Soldier and Biological Chemical Command (SBCCOM), *Guidelines for Mass Casualty Decontamination During a Terrorist Chemical Agent Incident*, ECBC-TR-125, January 2000.

In the case where forces are recovered and arrive via landing craft in the well deck, damage control crew can stage expedient showers using either the well deck sprinkler systems or fire hoses and fog nozzles to create mass showers, as recommended in Army guidelines for civilian emergency response.

If wind generated through the well deck exits from the aft section of the ship, the area forward of the well deck—which includes the lower vehicle area and the balance of the ship—is beyond the vapor hazard area. Medical department staff should meet recovered forces beyond the vapor hazard area to monitor their health and ensure that they are free of contaminants. Here, ships' crew can work free of protective gear, including gas masks, as long as there is no detectable vapor hazard present.

The Army guidelines recommend that approximately 100 persons per hour can process through an expedient shower area ten feet in width. By extension, a shower area three times that width that is established in the well deck of an amphibious assault ship can be conservatively estimated to process 300 service members in an hour.

Implementing expedient deck patient decontamination stations and expedient showers can increase ships' decontamination throughput from twelve litter patients per hour to 36 litter patients per hour, and from 60 ambulatory personnel per hour to 300 ambulatory personnel per hour.

What is the prognosis for connectors and ships returning to full military capability in support of the mission?

If contaminated patients are brought to existing patient decontamination stations, contaminants will be brought within the skin of the ship. When litter-bound casualties are decontaminated in expedient deck patient decontamination stations staged on the flight deck, contaminants are kept out of interior spaces. Ships' crews must be assured that CMWDS will effectively remove contaminates as quickly as they are capable.

Landing craft can generally be decontaminated more easily than aircraft. Selecting landing craft to recover contaminated forces can ease connector decontamination.

Will the ships be required to return to port for reconstitution?

Using CMWDS to remove contaminants from ships' exterior surfaces, and decontaminating interior spaces with high-test hypochlorite solution, ships' damage control crew can thoroughly decontaminate ships so that they can continue their mission without returning to port for decontamination. However, ships face a persistent threat of cross-contamination when recovered forces have been infected with biological agents. In order to remain at sea without returning to port to offload contagious passengers, ships must plan to isolate them from the uninfected crew. The Navy is able to manage biological hazards requiring standard and contact precautions using current medical department capabilities aboard amphibious ships. The precautions necessary to prevent cross-contamination for hazards requiring airborne precautions pose a challenge for

Navy ships. Options exist to prevent airborne biological hazard cross-contamination, which are discussed in further detail in the body of the report.

Conclusions

The Navy's capability to recover contaminated and injured forces to the sea base during amphibious missions is limited by two primary factors. The first is lack of an efficient process to evaluate the operational environment and identify connectors and ships based on transportation requirements for the recovery operation. The second is a limitation in the capacity and throughput to recover contaminated personnel onboard ships. To improve Navy capability, this study makes the following recommendations:

1. Develop a decision process for recovery operations. Once it is determined that contaminated forces will be recovered to the sea base, the operational commander must quickly decide which ship(s) will receive the contaminated forces and how the forces will be transported to the ship. These decisions are based largely on the number of forces to be recovered and the extent and nature of casualties. In addition, the requirements for and location of decontamination operations must be determined, with the primary goal of reducing the spread of contaminants.

2. Employ expedient deck decontamination processes aboard amphibious assault ships to increase personnel decontamination throughput per hour. Set up expedient patient decontamination stations on the flight deck and expedient showers in the well deck. Such a configuration will speed decontamination, minimize the areas where JSLIST gear must be worn, and decrease the time required to thoroughly decontaminate and return the ship to full military capability.

Implementing these recommendations will require some change in DOTMLPF (doctrine, organization, training, materiel, leadership and education, personnel, and facilities). Primarily, the Navy needs to amend doctrine to strengthen guidance in these areas, and train its forces to be familiar with and proficient at performing recovery operations. Minor changes are also needed to organization, materiel, and personnel. But overall, implementing these recommendations is well within the Navy's reach, as additional costs in terms of needed materiel and personnel are nominal.

The Navy has included operations to recover amphibious forces in CBR environments in recent tabletop exercises and in studies sponsored by RAND and CNA to address this mission (see McGrady, 2010). Isolating contagious service members has been studied at even greater length.[5] If the Navy incorporates such scenarios in its planning requirements, it could address its gaps in capability by implementing recommendations from this study.

---

[5] Joint Requirements Office for CBRN Defense, *Shipboard Isolation and Quarantine Concept Experiment Final Report*, May 2011, not available to the general public.

Acronyms

BUMED	Navy Bureau of Medicine and Surgery
CBR	chemical, biological, or radiological
CBRN	chemical, biological, radiological and nuclear
CBRNIAC	Chemical, Biological, Radiological and Nuclear Defense Information Analysis Center
CCA	contamination control area
C-HAG	Chemical Hazard Awareness Guide
CMWDS	Countermeasures Washdown System
COMSEC	Communications security
CPS	Collective Protection Systems
DOTMLPF	doctrine, organization, training, materiel, leadership and education, personnel, and facilities
ESG	Expeditionary Strike Group
HEPA	high-efficiency particulate air
HMMWVs	high mobility multipurpose wheeled vehicles
HTH	high-test hypochlorite
ICAMs	Improved Chemical Agent Monitors
JBPDS	Joint Biological Point Detection System
JSLIST	Joint Service Lightweight Integrated Suit Technology
LCAC	Landing Craft Air Cushion
LCU	Landing Craft Utility
LHA	Landing Helicopter Assault
LHD	Landing Helicopter Dock

LPD	Landing Platform Dock
LSD	Landing Ship Dock
M/cas-COAT	Medical/Casualty Course of Action Tool
MCESS	Marine Corps Expeditionary Shelter System
MEU	Marine Expeditionary Unit
MTTP	multiservice tactics, techniques, and procedures
NDRI	National Defense Research Institute
NSTM	Naval Ships' Technical Manual
NSWCCD	Naval Surface Warfare Center, Carderock Division
NWDC	Navy Warfare Development Command
NTTP	Navy tactics, techniques, and procedures
PDS	patient decontamination station
PTM	Personnel Transport Module
ROC and POE	Required Operational Capabilities and Projected Operational Environment
RSDL	reactive self-decontamination lotion
SBCCOM	Soldier and Biological Chemical Command
SWOS	Surface Warfare Officer's School

1. Introduction

The mission to recover amphibious forces can be complicated if ashore forces come under attack from enemy weapons, particularly chemical, biological, or radiological (CBR) weapons. If ashore forces are attacked with CBR weapons, they may become contaminated and pose a cross-contamination risk to other forces with whom they come in contact. If contaminants spread to equipment and vehicles, creating persistent hazards, these items may pose an additional cross-contamination risk. Among the potential agents that may be used in CBR weapons, persistent liquid and solid chemical agents present the greatest challenge for physical decontamination.

Navy military capability will be compromised when ships' resources are dedicated to recover contaminated ashore forces. The personnel dedicated to the recovery mission will be redirected away from their primary responsibilities. Areas of ships used in the recovery mission will be unusable for other activities during the recovery process and for the duration until they are determine free of any potential contaminants. Navy capability will be further degraded as personnel who are injured by the CBR agents become casualties, and as casualties with conventional injuries become contaminated with CBR agents that exacerbate their underlying medical conditions.

In 2010, a series of tabletop exercises[6] conducted by the Navy revealed specific issues in Navy doctrine and capabilities related to transporting contaminated forces from land to the sea base and decontaminating contaminated forces aboard ships. Participants in the exercise expressed concern that the Navy lacked clearly defined capabilities to recover contaminated forces. Issues of concern included:

1. *Which amphibious assault ship should receive contaminated forces*? Each ship in the battle group has different decontamination and medical department capabilities, which must be well understood before recovery decisions are made.
2. *Which connector is best to go ashore and bring forces back to the sea base?* Air and sea craft may be contaminated while recovering ashore forces. Therefore, it is necessary to determine whether a landing craft air cushion (LCAC), landing craft utility (LCU), or aircraft (and which model of aircraft) can best withstand contamination as well as return the forces quickly and safely.
3. *What procedures should be used to decontaminate the forces when they arrive aboard the ships?* Forces should be decontaminated quickly so that their conditions do not worsen, and the spread of contaminants throughout the ship should be minimized.
4. *What is the prognosis for connectors and ships returning to full military capability in support of the mission?* Decontamination procedures should be

[6] Navy Craft CBRN Survivability tabletop exercises, August 2010.

managed to maximize ships' ability to maintain and return to fully military capability.
5. *Will the ships be required to return to port for reconstitution?* Or can ships remain at sea to continue the mission?

In order to address the capabilities identified in these exercises, researchers from RAND National Defense Research Institute (NDRI) were contracted by OPNAV N81 to assess current policies and capabilities pertaining to the recovery and decontamination of ashore forces, and to identify policy options the Navy could pursue to better perform this mission. RAND designed a study addressing the Navy capabilities required to perform the following amphibious mission functions:

- Transport contaminated and injured forces from shore to ship
- Decontaminate and treat litter-bound casualties at the sea base
- Decontaminate ambulatory and uninjured forces
- Return ships and transports to full mission capability.

This research develops a set of policies to increase the Navy's capability to recover and transport contaminated land forces to amphibious assault groups. It also proposes doctrine to support operational decisions. It is crucial that the Navy have doctrinally defined procedures supported with capability enablers, such as proper training and materiel, to achieve optimal mission outcomes. This report includes policy recommendations for the Navy to pursue along the joint capability development spectrum of doctrine, organization, training, materiel, leadership and education, personnel, and facilities (DOTMLPF).

Study Scope

Interviews with Navy damage control and Marine Corps CBR staff members suggested that to maintain the capability of ashore forces and to avoid spreading contaminants to the sea base, the preference would be to decontaminate forces ashore. If it is not feasible to decontaminate ashore forces in the operating environment, the next-preferred option would be to move the forces to a clean area where it would be safe to perform operational decontamination, exchange protective gear, and return the forces to duty. Based on these recommendations, the Navy should only consider recovering contaminated forces to the sea base when it is infeasible to decontaminate ashore.

This study is based on the assumption that thorough decontamination facilities ashore and in transit are not available. Therefore, the study focused on the mission to transport, recover, and decontaminate forces. (Transporting casualties is addressed briefly in this document. Medical treatment of casualties en route and the effect of CBR injuries on the demand for medical care at the sea base or after evacuation out of theater were not addressed.

In project interviews, Navy CBR staff indicated that they would only consider recovering materiel that was security-sensitive. This position is consistent with guidance in draft document Navy Tactics, Techniques, and Procedures (NTTP) 3-02.1.1M:

Decontamination priorities should be established prior to beginning recovery operations. Although every situation has unique characteristics, the following priorities should be considered as a guide:

1. Personnel
2. Sensitive equipment (e.g., communications security (COMSEC))
3. Combat-essential equipment and supplies
4. Other equipment and supplies.

Recovering contaminated materiel is not analyzed in this study.

Assumptions

The analysis is structured around a broad set of assumptions in order to ensure that the recommendations are applicable across future Navy planning scenarios. To make the scope less expansive, the analysis was refined to include only connectors and ships well-suited to recovering contaminated forces in amphibious missions. This limits the ships only to those that contain onboard medical capabilities and are of sufficient size to recover an adequate number of personnel.

Navy staff responsible for capability planning confirmed that the scenarios are both realistic with respect to Navy resources involved with the mission, and stressing with the number of forces assumed contaminated and injured.

Ships

The study design includes recovery to an amphibious assault group composed of Landing Helicopter Dock (LHD), Landing Platform Dock (LPD), and Landing Ship Dock (LSD) ships. With only one Landing Helicopter Assault (LHA) remaining in the active fleet, the study does not address the LHA. The LPD-17, San Antonio class, is addressed in the study because it has capabilities beyond older classes of LPD.

Interviews with damage control and medical department staff working on amphibious assault ships showed that ships smaller than amphibious assault ships are not feasible for recovery. Lack of well decks to receive landing craft precludes recovering large numbers of forces in amphibious missions. Additionally, smaller ships, such as destroyers and frigates, have minimal medical assets, making them less capable to treat casualties of any magnitude. In missions where contaminated forces are recovered to the sea base, it is assumed that forces requiring medical attention will be expected.

Connectors

The following connectors were analyzed in the recovery mission: CH-46 Sea Knight, CH-53E Sea Stallion, MV-22 Osprey, Landing Craft Air Cushion (LCAC), Landing Craft Utility (LCU). These connectors are carried by amphibious assault ships and possess passenger-carrying capability.

Scenario Specifics

The study assumes that the battle group is 15 nautical miles off shore—a typical distance for Navy battle groups.[7] At this distance, connectors are within range to provide support to forces ashore.

Ashore Forces—Population at Risk

The study assumed that the ashore force is a Marine Expeditionary Unit (MEU). A MEU consists of approximately 3,000 Marines, 1,000 Marines in each amphibious assault ship. Therefore, it is assumed that the maximum number of forces that would deploy ashore (population at risk) is 3,000. In scenarios where a larger ashore population is attacked by an enemy CBR weapon, it was assumed that the ashore forces should have land-based support.

The study assumed that 10 percent of ashore forces are contaminated, requiring recovery for decontamination. This is a robust upper bound on the number of forces requiring evacuation and decontamination. It is consistent with the capacity the Army supplies its infantry to decontaminate personnel (see FM 4-02.7/NTTP 4-02.7). The study also assumed that up to 3 percent of the total ashore forces are wounded in action with conventional injuries (that may be exacerbated by contamination). This rate is higher than casualty rates estimated for similar missions using the Medical/Casualty Course of Action Tool (M/Cas-COAT). M/Cas-COAT is an Army tool that generates casualty estimates.[8] To provide a taxing scenario, the study assumed an upper bound of 24 litter-bound casualties. Twenty-four litter-bound casualties is consistent with the limit on litter passengers on a CH-53E.[9] In total, the study assumed the maximum contaminated and injured population to be

---

[7] When interviewed, a LHD Damage Control Assistant indicated that in scenarios where the CBR enemy attack is a potential, a distance of 15 nm offshore would be reasonable for analysis. In subsequent interviews, Navy damage control personnel concurred with this assumption.

[8] The M/Cas-COAT is unclassified and generates casualty estimates based on such factors as type of unit (operational or support), terrain, weather, size of unit, combat effectiveness, equipment superiority, and others.

[9] Department of the Navy, Office of the Chief of Naval Operations, and Headquarters, U.S. Marine Corps, *Ship-to-Shore Movement*, NWP 3-02.1/MCWP 3-31.5, August 1993.

- 300 total contaminated service members, including
- 24 contaminated litter casualties, and
- 75 contaminated ambulatory casualties.

All forces required to return to the sea base were assumed to have some contaminant on them that is external to intact protective gear, has penetrated through protective gear, or is directly on unprotected skin and garments. In any case, the recovered forces must undergo thorough decontamination in order to be allowed into the interior of the ship. Upon returning to the sea base, medical department staff should triage the recovered forces. To expedite treatment, those with urgent and emergent conditions should be decontaminated first. As long as the objective is to recover, decontaminate, and treat recovered forces quickly, the policies recommended should apply broadly.

Research Approach

The study research approach included gathering data through a literature review and interviews with subject matter experts. Using these data, the study identified the Navy's current capability to perform the recovery and decontamination activities described previously and proposed solutions to increase Navy capability for these defined amphibious mission functions. The full set of documents reviewed for this study is listed in the reference section. Interviews were conducted with staff from the following organizations: OPNAV N86; Navy Bureau of Medicine and Surgery (BUMED) CBR research; Navy Warfare Development Command (NWDC); Marine Corps CBRN; LHD/LPD damage control; LHD flight deck and well deck operations; fleet surgical team; Afloat Training Group; Assault Craft Unit; Naval Surface Warfare Center, Carderock Division (NSWCCD) damage control engineering; Third Fleet; Naval Surface Forces; Pacific Fleet; Surface Warfare Officer School–CBR training; Chemical, Biological, Radiological and Nuclear Defense Information Analysis Center (CBRNIAC); and Los Angeles County Public Health.

Current Navy processes to decontaminate forces were documented on the basis of current military guidance and interviews with service members. Some aspects of current Navy capability to recover contaminated forces in amphibious environments were identified by reporting quantitative data found in current military documents, such as the time until chemical agents dissipate from the surface of Navy ships. Other measures of capability, such as the time necessary to transport contaminated forces from shore to ship using each of the connectors in the study, were calculated using basic spreadsheet models populated with numerical data derived from current guidance, Navy damage control crew interviews, and basic assumptions. No operational tests of capability were performed in this study.

The companion report, RR-155/1, includes data and analysis identifying the current capability of ships' medical departments to treat casualties at sea in order to better understand the extent to which medical department throughput constrains overall Navy capability to recover forces. However, opportunities to increase the capability of ships' medical departments, and implications for medical treatment of casualties en route (during evacuation) were not considered.

The study addressed the Navy objective to recover all required forces and maintain battle group capability. To achieve this goal, the study recommends options to increase capability and projects the burden of decontaminating connectors and ships. Resources dedicated to recovery and decontamination missions will be unavailable to other missions and therefore come with an opportunity cost. Resources may also be unavailable for a longer duration if they become contaminated during the recovery mission, requiring additional time to decontaminate or reconstitute. Based on an understanding of these implications, the researchers were able to project the net effect of recovery operations on battle groups. Operational tests of technologies or procedures were not performed.

2. Current Navy Processes

The study reviewed current Navy processes to recover contaminated forces in amphibious missions (Appendix A). Extant military guidance, both Navy and multi-service, was referenced, including one draft document that is intended to be the authoritative guidance for recovering forces in CBR environments—NTTP 3-02.1.1M, *Recovery Operations in a Chemical, Biological, Radiological and Nuclear (CBRN) Environment*. According to this guidance, forces should be decontaminated before returning to the ship, if possible. NTTP 3-20.31[10] should be referred to for additional details about how ships should individually prepare for CBR attacks, and how plans should be documented in ships' CBR Defense Bills.

As mentioned in the previous chapter, prior to deciding to recover contaminated forces to the sea base, the Navy should consider whether options are available to decontaminate forces ashore, according to the decision process detailed in Figure 2.1.

[10] Department of the Navy, Office of the Chief of Naval Operations, *Surface Ship Survivability*, NTTP 3-20.31/COMDTINST M3440.1, 15 August 2011.

Figure 2.1 Decision Process to Recover Contaminated Forces

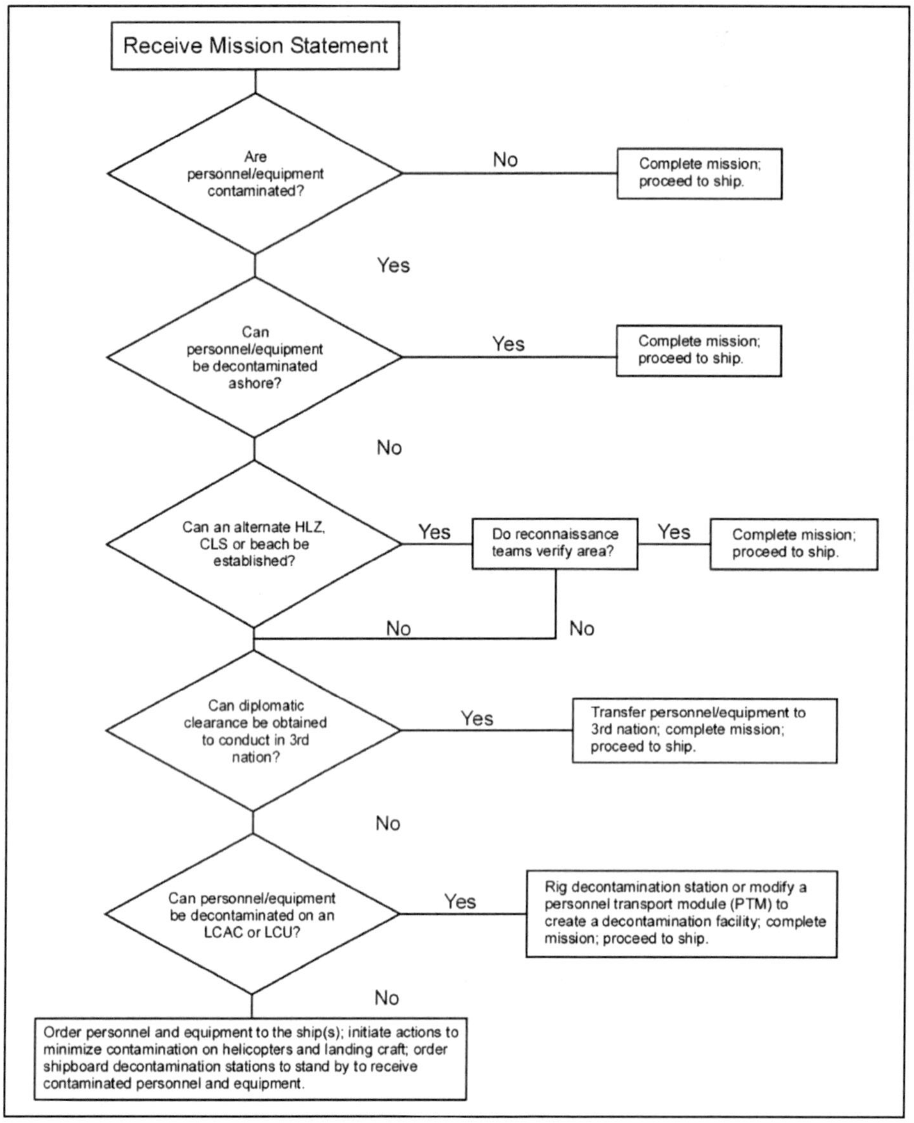

SOURCE: NTTP 3-02.1.1M.

If MEU personnel and equipment are contaminated during a mission and personnel cannot be decontaminated ashore, forces would be recovered and transported to the sea base. Complete decontamination involves personnel, connectors, and ships, as described in the remainder of this chapter.

Decontaminate Personnel

The Navy provides its ships with equipment capable of detecting the presence of chemical hazards and has plans to deliver equipment to detect biological hazards. Navy ships carry outfits to protect service members against chemical and biological hazards. These outfits are referred to as Joint Service Lightweight Integrated Suit Technology (JSLIST) gear, which consists of a protective mask, overgarment, boots, and gloves.

Navy ships included in this study have collective protection systems (CPS), which are ventilation systems providing full protection from CBR agents to areas of the ship that are within protected zones. In the protected zones, all CBR contaminants are filtered from incoming air, and positive pressure is maintained so that no air enters the zone through other routes. To enter and exit the zones, ships' crew members must pass through air locks. When in the protected zones, crew members do not need to wear protective gear, such as outer garments or masks.

Navy guidance describes three stages of decontamination:

- Immediate decontamination
- Operational decontamination
- Thorough decontamination.

Immediate Decontamination

NTTP 3-11.26[11] contains specific guidance for recovering contaminated forces to the sea base. Preferable methods of decontamination of personnel are as follow:

1. For liquid-transmitted chemical agents, the M291 Skin Decontamination Kit is the first choice to remove and neutralize a contaminant. A second choice is to blot the liquid contaminant, and flush the skin area with water, and soap if it is available. For aerosol and vapor transmitted chemical agents, soap and water is the preferred method to decontaminate.
2. For biological agents, soap and water are used to remove nearly all agents from skin. A solution of 0.5 percent high-test hypochlorite (HTH) is also an effective decontaminant.
3. For radiological agents, brushing or wiping off the physical contaminant is quite effective. In cases where contaminant may remain, washing with soap and water should be performed.

---

[11] Department of the Navy, *Multiservice Tactics, Techniques, and Procedures for Chemical, Biological, Radiological, and Nuclear Decontamination*, FM 3-11.5/MCWP 3-37.3/NTTP 3-11.26/AFTTP(I) 3-2.60 IX-13, 2006.

Patient Decontamination

FM 4-02.7[12] defines immediate patient decontamination:

> Immediate (Patient): Complete decontamination of contaminated areas of patient's MOPP prior to evacuation or RTD, without removing MOPP.

This decontamination is to be performed as self-aid or buddy aid.

Operational Decontamination

To perform operational decontamination, service members move to uncontaminated areas, remove contaminated but intact JSLIST gear, and don uncontaminated JSLIST gear. Performing this procedure allows service members rest and respite from the heat that may build up while wearing JSLIST gear and allows forces to continue their duties in a contaminated environment.

Patient Decontamination

According to FM 4-02.7 operational patient decontamination is not defined in a way that is distinguishable from thorough patient decontamination.

> Operational/Thorough (Patient): Decontamination at a [patient decontamination station] PDS and treatment of conventional and chemical injuries at MTF prior to transport using ground, water, and air.

This decontamination should be performed by medical department augmentees and supervised by medical department personnel.

`Thorough Decontamination

NSTM Chapter 470 directs that personnel decontamination should be performed in five stages:

1. Remove outer-gear and perform gross decontamination of masks, boots, and gloves. Gross decontamination of outer-gear is performed with M291 kits, or a calcium hypochlorite solution.
2. Remove over-garment.
3. Remove inner clothing.
4. Shower and remove CPS mask if in an area free of vapor hazards.
5. A member of the medical staff screens for symptoms of agent exposure and other medical problems such as heat stress. Patients must be decontaminated before medical treatment is begun. However, certain lifesaving procedures should be performed as soon as possible.

---

[12] Department of the Navy, *Multiservice Tactics, Techniques, and Procedures for Health Service Support in a Chemical, Biological, Radiological, and Nuclear Environment*, FM 4-02.7/MCRP 4-1.1F/NTTP 4-02.7/AFTTP 3-42.3, 2009.

Some ships have dedicated decontamination stations that provide areas where personnel decontamination can be performed while limiting risk of hazardous runoff or cross-contamination to other areas of the ship. NSTM Chapter 470 includes diagrams of dedicated areas in which service members may process through step 1 of the decontamination process, and then steps 2–5 (Figures 2.2 and 2.3).

Figure 2.2 Contamination Control Area for Decontamination Step 1[13]

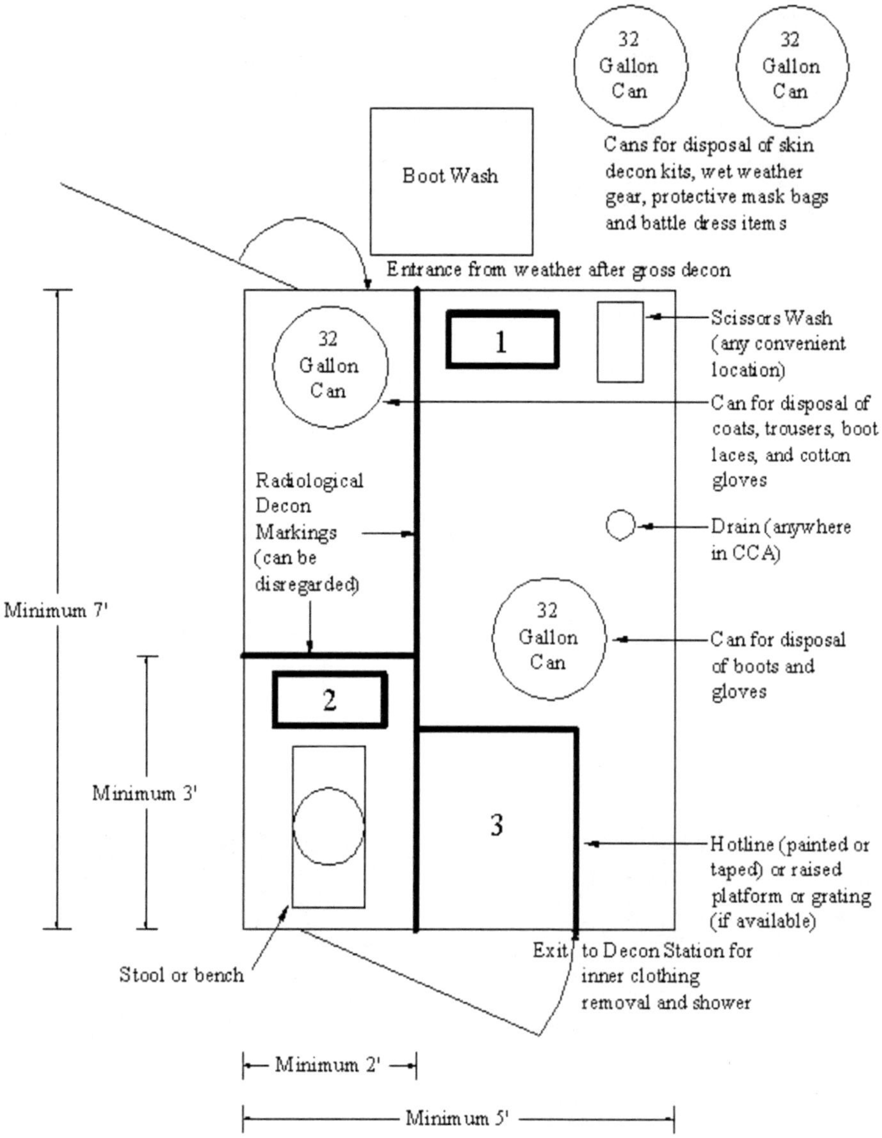

[13] *Naval Ships' Technical Manual*, Chapter 470, 2006b.

Figure 2.3 Contamination Control Area for Decontamination Steps 2–5[14]

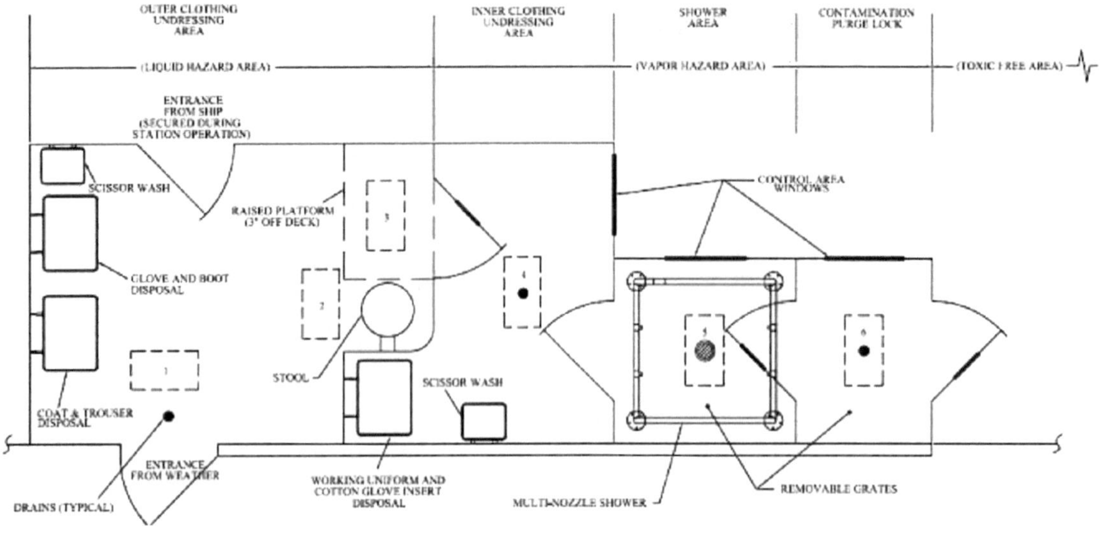

These dedicated contamination control and decontamination areas are designed for ambulatory personnel who remain upright throughout the disrobing and showering processes. The Navy has also outfitted some of its ships with decontamination stations suitable to process litter patients (Figure 2.4).

Figure 2.4 Patient Decontamination Station[15]

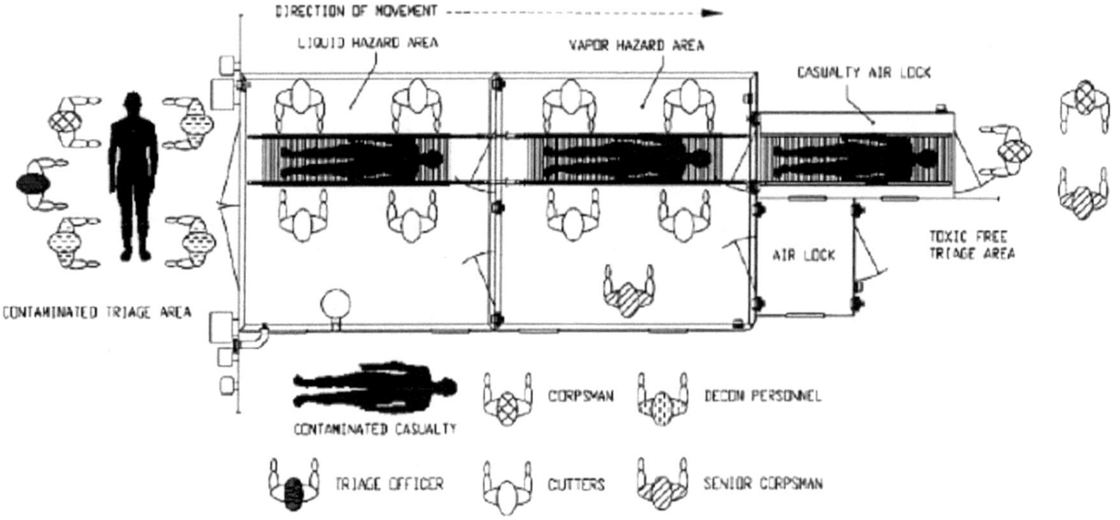

---

[14] *Naval Ships' Technical Manual,* Chapter 470, 2006b.

[15] *Naval Ships' Technical Manual*, Chapter 470, 2006b.

Patient decontamination stations include three compartments. Prior to entering the first compartment, injured service members should have their contaminated outer gear removed, as in step 1 of personnel decontamination. In the first compartment, litter bearers or other ships crew remove the patients' outer clothing, as in step 2 of personnel decontamination. In the second compartment, inner garments are removed, and the patient is rinsed, as in steps 3 and 4 of personnel decontamination. In the third chamber, the airlock, patients wait for two to three minutes[16] to ensure that all vapor hazards are purged. Then they are free to exit in the collective protection shelter of the ship and remove their masks.

There are five options a Navy ship can use to provide showers for personnel decontamination. One option is to use established personnel decontamination stations. The other four options offer methods to decontaminate ambulatory and uninjured service members that can supplement existing decontamination stations. The five options are

1. *Established decontamination showers*. Showers offer the best facility to complete personal decontamination. The ship's decontamination teams can monitor personnel through view ports, and contaminated personnel can be guided in completing the required procedures.
2. *Locally manufactured showers*. Locally manufactured showers offer the flexibility to meet the design variations within classes of ships, assist in overcoming shortfalls in decontamination station locations and quantities, and complement locally developed plans to process individuals with varying needs.
3. *Portable shower tents*. Portable shower tents offer flexibility for decontaminating a large force or group of civilians. Easy to erect, these portable and self-contained units include all the piping and wastewater containment capability required to complement a contamination control area (CCA).
4. *Field showers from embarked units*. Field showers, designed and utilized by forces ashore, are another option to meet the challenge of decontaminating a large number of personnel. This equipment most likely would be sent to the field in support of the landing force or naval support elements, and will be an essential part of the effort to complete their decontamination prior to retrograding to the ship. The ship's use of such equipment will require a memorandum of understanding to be established in advance of such operations.
5. *Fire hoses*. Rigging fire hoses to create a makeshift shower serves as a minimal resource for providing a shower to retrograding personnel.[17]

After completing these processes, personnel are monitored for residual contamination by corpsmen or medical department crew members. Service members are monitored for radiological contamination with a RADIAC.[18] If service members are observed to have no more than ambient levels of contamination and show no symptoms requiring medical

[16] Per interviews with amphibious assault ship damage control crew.

[17] FM 3-11.5/MCWP 3-37.3/NTTP 3-11.26/AFTTP(I) 3-2.60 IX-13, April 2006.

[18] RADIAC is a device used for radiation detection, indication, and computation.

attention, they can be allowed to proceed to their quarters where they can continue showering if any contamination remains.

For chemical contamination, service members are monitored with M8/M9 paper or improved chemical agent monitors (ICAMs). If no residual contamination is found and service members show no concerning symptoms, they are considered thoroughly decontaminated.

The Joint Biological Point Detection System (JBPDS) biological hazard monitoring equipment has been installed on some, but not all amphibious assault ships. This equipment is being continually studied for effectiveness and improvements. Additional biological capability aboard amphibious assault ships includes manual collection and identification; a process which may take several hours. When forces are recovered to the sea base, and are concerned that they may have come under attack from a weapon that released biological agents, the service members should process through soap and water decontamination by patient decontamination stations or showers in order to ensure all solid contaminants are removed. If service members appear to have symptoms of infection from biological agents, they should be examined by medical department staff and have specimens collected for ships[1] laboratories to determine whether they are infected.

Table 2.1 contains a comprehensive list of decontamination procedures for each type of CBR agent. In cases where persistent liquid or solid chemical agents are used against ashore forces, the risk of residual contamination is greater than with other agents; such agents require urgent, thorough decontamination to minimize the risk of injury and cross-contamination of other personnel and surfaces. By contrast, personnel can be largely freed of radioactive material by shaking outer garments, or brushing off residue. In all cases, washing or showering is effective for thorough personnel decontamination.

Table 2.1 Decontamination Techniques for CBR Agents

Type of Application	*Type of Contaminant*					
	Chemical		*Biological*		*Nuclear/Radiological*	
Decontaminants/Techniques	**Personnel: (immediate and time critical)**	**Surface/ Material/Area**	**Personnel: (not time critical)**	**Surface/ Material/Area**	**Personnel: (less time critical)**	**Surface/ Material/ Area**
Misting hair/clothes	minimize reaerosolization		minimize reaerosolization		minimize reaerosolization	
Physical removal	remove outer garments		remove outer garments		dry brushing/shaking	dry brushing/ shaking
Water only	X	X	X			
Soap and Water	X	X	X	X	X	X
Weathering		X		X		X
Skin Decontamination	X		X			
Individual Equipment Decontamination Kit		equipment		equipment		
STB/HTH		X*		X*		
M100 SDS reactive powder		X*		X*		X
Household bleach solution (5% sodium hypochlorite)		X*		X*		
Dilute bleach solution (0.5% sodium hypochlorite)	^	X	^	X		
Absorbents (earth/soil, sawdust, ashes, rags)		for liquid decon				
Sealants/physical covers (concrete, asphalt, paint, soil)		X		X		X
Steam		§		X		X
Heat/Fire/Incineration		X		X		

* These particularly corrosive decontaminants are specifically not to be used on certain aircraft and other equipment (a soap and water alternative is doctrinally mandated. See FM 3-11.5/MCWP 3-37.3/NTTP 3-11.26/AFTTP(I) 3-2.60 for more details.

^ While military doctrine allows this for decon of persons, federal guidance stipulates that only water or soap and water should be used for personnel/mass decon. See *Best Practice Guidelines for CBR Mass Personnel Decontamination*, 2004.

§ Steam, as well as certain vaporized gases (ammonia, hydrogen peroxide, chlorine dioxide) may be used for the decontamination of interior buildings/heating, ventilation, and air conditioning. These can be logistically involved operations. See hazard chapters of above-mentioned guidelines for specific subject matter expert support.

SOURCE: NTTP 4-02.7.

Decontaminate Connectors

Inherent in the mission to recover forces to the sea base are the choice and use of a connector. Connectors are aircraft or ships used to transport forces from the shore to the ship. Connectors may become contaminated by landing in a contaminated area or as a result of cross-contamination from the transport of contaminated forces.

Certain classes of landing craft have the ability to self-decontaminate with specified procedures. Landing craft may also position themselves near larger ships, such as amphibious assault ships, where saltwater fire hoses may be trained upon the landing craft to remove contaminants.

LCUs have a Countermeasures Washdown System (CMWDS), a set of sprinklers the crafts' crew members can activate to remove contaminant from the exterior of the craft prior to arriving at the sea base. The procedures to perform LCU decontamination are described in NTTP 3-11.26:

> The LCU initiates active decontamination during transit to the ship, including activation of its CMWDS. Upon nearing the ship, the LCU should be directed to take and maintain its station alongside the ship at the slowest and safest possible speed. Once alongside, the ship's force uses additional fire hoses from the catwalks to concentrate on those areas not fully covered by the LCU system. The LCU crew is then directed to survey their exterior and report results to the ship; any hot spots will be further decontaminated. If agents have been left on the craft for over an hour, the epoxy-based paint may have absorbed them and a thorough decontamination may be required. The ship's force and LCU crews should pay particular attention to the crew cabin ventilation, air conditioning systems, and the large filter units for the engine air intake system. The crew cabin ventilation system can create a serious vapor hazard by blowing the agent vapor into an otherwise sealed compartment.

LCACs can perform a "bird bath" procedure in which propellers are reversed and the craft proceeds down and across the wind. This procedure is an effective way to remove contaminants from the exterior of LCACs. Procedures for decontaminating LCACs are also described in NTTP 3-11.26:

> The craftmasters shall maneuver their craft to maximize the exposure to sea spray. Propeller reversal, with the craft proceeding downwind and across the wind, is recommended as a minimum. If the craftmaster's survey confirms that the craft is clean, direct the craft to proceed into the well. Conversely, if the craft is still contaminated and the tactical situation and sea state permit, direct the LCAC to go off-cushion astern or alongside the ship. Have the ship's well deck crew hose down the craft with saltwater from the stern or catwalks; avoid hitting the LCAC propellers with a solid stream of water.

The challenge of decontaminating LCACs is greater if the craft travels over land, through a contaminated area. If the LCAC travels over land to recover or deliver its load, contaminants will have been absorbed into permeable material, presenting a long-lasting contact and vapor hazard. At-risk material includes nonskid coverings and the rubber skirt; a thorough decontamination will likely result in their removal and replacement.

Aircraft decontamination is time-consuming and difficult to perform. Currently, there are no available decontamination technologies other than using standard aircraft soaps and cleaners to displace contamination from aircraft. When aircraft are finished flying missions that have contamination risk, it is recommended that they be washed down to remove contaminants. When performing washdown, aircraft should be located as far aft on the flight deck as possible, behind the superstructure on large-deck ships, so they are positioned downwind from other areas of the ship. Spot decontamination, including washing aircraft surfaces with sponges or rags, may also be required.

The challenge of thoroughly decontaminating aircraft is compounded because contamination may reach throughout aircraft systems and subsystems that are confined behind panels and access hatches. Contamination may reach into aircraft components, which should be sent to maintenance activities to be processed rather than treated locally aboard Navy ships. If significant contamination reaches the interior or internal areas of an aircraft, it will certainly require hours of effort to perform an aircraft washdown, after which contamination may still remain.

Decontaminate Ships

Ships are decontaminated with their CMWDS, a set of sprinklers designed to thoroughly wet down all weather decks and the superstructure, and to produce sufficient runoff of water to remove contaminants. Hot spots are manually scrubbed.

3. Current Navy Capability

The assessment of current Navy capability is structured around the following mission functions:

- Transport contaminated and injured forces from shore to ship
- Decontaminate and treat litter-bound casualties at the sea base
- Decontaminate ambulatory and uninjured forces
- Return ships and connectors to full mission capability.

Each of these functions is discussed in detail in the remainder of this chapter.

Transport Contaminated and Injured Forces from Shore to Ship

The connectors included in this study range in capacity to carry litter and ambulatory passengers, and in speed (Table 3.1). The capacity to carry litter passengers ranges from 15 passengers in a CH-46 to 100 in an LCU. Similarly, capacity for ambulatory passengers ranges from 22 to 400. The time to transport also differs by connector, ranging from 7 minutes per 15 nautical miles for a CH-46 to over 80 minutes for an LCU.

Table 3.1 Capability of Navy Connectors[19]

	Litter Passengers	Ambulatory Passengers	Minutes / 15 nm
MV-22	12	24	3
CH-46	15	22	7
CH-53E	24	52	6
LCAC: Passenger Configured	110	220	23
LCU	100	400	82

In Table 3.1, the capacity of connectors to carry both litter-bound and ambulatory passengers are not additive. If a connector carries a combination of litter and ambulatory passengers, its capacity will be proportionate to the quantity of each type of passenger aboard. LCACs have limited passenger space in their cabins. Forces generally travel aboard LCACs by riding in hard-topped vehicles such as High Mobility Multipurpose

[19] Department of the Navy, *Ship to Shore Movement*, NWP 3-02.1, 1993.

Wheeled Vehicles (HMMWVs) that are secured to the LCAC deck. The LCAC's passenger-carrying capability is greatly increased when it is outfitted with a set such as a Marine Corps Expeditionary Shelter System (MCESS) or a Personnel Transport Module (PTM),[20] in which large numbers of forces may ride safely.

Using the data in Table 3.1, and basic assumptions about the time required to load and unload connectors, the time required to recover forces using each of the connectors and total passenger throughput can be calculated. In order to assess current Navy capability, it is assumed that connectors are loaded in fifteen minutes and unloaded in five minutes. Policy options included in the following section are not sensitive to this assumption. Connectors are assumed to originate from the sea base. To estimate the time to recover forces in an operational setting, these factors can be adjusted, as can the battle group distance from shore. The formulas to calculate the times and rates listed in Table 3.2 are as follows:

*Time to Recover Passengers = 2 * (Minutes / 15 nm) + Time to Load Connector + Time to Unload Connector*

*Passengers Recovered per Hour = (60 / Time to Recover Passengers) * Connector Passengers*

Table 3.2 Time to Recover Passengers and Connector Throughput

Connector	Time to Recover Passengers, One Sortie (minutes)	Passengers Recovered per Hour Litter : Ambulatory
MV-22	26	28 : 55
CH-46	34	26 : 39
CH-53E	32	45 : 98
LCAC: Passenger Configured	66	100 : 200
LCU	184	33 : 130

NOTE: Passengers recovered per hour are not additive. Connectors can recover either the indicated number of litter or ambulatory passengers, or a proportionate combination.

[20] Shelters are comparable in size to a 20-foot shipping container, of which the Navy has a limited inventory.

Decontaminate and Treat Litter-Bound Casualties at the Sea Base

Of the ships included in this study, LHD-1 and LPD-17 have patient decontamination stations (sometimes referred to as medical or casualty decontamination stations). It takes approximately five minutes to process a contaminated and injured service member through each of the first two compartments of a patient decontamination station. Patients must spend two to three minutes in the third compartment to allow the airlock to purge any remaining vapor hazards.[21] At this rate, if the crew manning patient decontamination stations is efficient, both ships can process twelve patients per hour (Table 3.3).

Table 3.3 Patient Decontamination Capability

Ship	Patient Decontamination Stations	Patients Decontaminated per Hour
LHD-1	1	12
LPD-17	1	12
LPD-4, LSD	0	0

The two ship types with patient decontamination capability, LHD-1 and LPD-17, are the same two types with medical departments capable of performing surgeries.[22] Data and analysis assessing the capability of these ships to receive patients are included in an FOUO version of this document, RR-155/1-OSD, which is available upon request from RAND NSRD.

In order to receive patients at the planned rates, ships' medical departments must be supplemented beyond their organic staffing, to include a fleet surgical team, of which there may be only one deployed with an amphibious assault group.[23] This team is composed of three medical officers (including one general surgeon), three nurses, and nine corpsmen. The fleet surgical team is typically stationed on the large-deck amphibious assault ship, the LHD, because it has the largest and most capable medical department of the amphibious assault group.

---

[21] Per interviews with amphibious assault ship damage control crew.

[22] Department of the Navy, *Contingency Fact Book*, 2006a.

[23] Amphibious assault group medical staff may be supplemented by more than one fleet surgical team during a deployment, but Navy documents do not include data describing such an augmentation or what capability it would present. MEU medical staff may also supplement ships' medical capabilities. But they may be unavailable as their primary mission is attending to service members in the Marine Corps units, and they may go ashore.

Decontaminate Ambulatory and Uninjured Forces

When recovering contaminated forces, damage control crew members are trained to bring the forces through established decontamination stations. Large-deck amphibious assault ships, such as LHD-1, have two such stations that enable forces to decontaminate and exit into the CPS. Small-deck amphibious assault ships, such as LPD-17, have one such station (Table 3.4). Ambulatory and uninjured forces can process through the disrobing and showering sections of conventional decontamination stations (see Figure 2.2) more quickly than litter patients through patient decontamination stations. However, two to three minutes are still required for service members to process through the airlock in the third compartment, to ensure that vapor hazards have been purged. At this rate, it is estimated that 30 service members per hour may process through these stations.

Table 3.4 Personnel Decontamination Capability

Ship	Decontamination Stations Exiting to CPS	Persons Decontaminated per Hour
LHD-1	2	60
LPD-17	1	30

Return Connectors and Ships to Full Mission Capability

When selecting a ship to receive contaminated forces, and connectors to transport the forces from shore to the sea base, a battle group commander must consider the opportunity cost of committing these resources to the mission. Crew members working in areas of ships and connectors that become contaminated must wear JSLIST gear, which impedes their abilities and requires them to take rests to avoid heat exhaustion. Ships and connectors have differing capabilities to decontaminate while at sea, which affect the time crew must wear protective gear.

Connectors

Both of the landing craft considered in this study have established procedures for removing contaminants from their external surfaces, as described in the previous chapter. But no data exist to estimate the time required to perform these decontamination procedures. This is also the case for aircraft used as transports. Prospects for decontaminating landing craft and aircraft are listed in Table 3.5.

Table 3.5 Prospects to Decontaminate Connectors

Connector	Thorough Decontamination Procedures	Confidence to Perform Quickly
LCU	During transit, activate CMWDS.	High
LCAC	Craftmasters maneuver craft to maximize exposure to sea spray (birdbath).	High
LCAC	If traveled over contaminated land, skirt may need to be removed and replaced.	Low
General landing craft	With landing craft alongside amphibious assault ship, ship's forces hoses down craft with seawater.	High
Aircraft: exterior	Apply warm, soapy water to exterior of aircraft.	High
Aircraft: interior	Spot decontaminate with rags dipped in warm, soapy water or other approved aircraft cleaner.	Low
Aircraft: systems	Turn over to emergency reclamation teams.	Low

Ships

Ships' CMWDS use sprinklers to spray water over external surfaces, including flight decks, superstructures, and catwalks. Liquid chemical hazards are the persistent hazards that remain on ships' surfaces; they can be removed effectively by CMWDS. When CMWDS are used to pre-wet surfaces in advance of CBR weapon attacks, the time to thoroughly remove contaminants is reduced. CMWDS may be similarly effective removing contaminants carried by recovered forces or connectors. The time required to fully remove contaminants varies by type of chemical hazard.

In scenarios where ashore forces are recovered to the sea base, ships' crew should have sufficient time to perform a pre-wet with the CMWDS. Doing so can reduce the time required to decontaminate ships' decks by 75 percent. When pre-wet, decks can be fully decontaminated within several hours for V type agents—even more quickly for H type blister and G type nerve agents (Tables 3.6–3.8). Depending on weather conditions, decks can be fully decontaminated from H blister and G nerve agents in as little time as 20 minutes, quickly returning the affected areas to use by unprotected personnel.

Table 3.6 V-Nerve Agents: Time to Decontaminate Ships' Decks

Countermeasure Washdown (CMWD) Situation	Estimated Deck Temperature		
	30°F	60°F	90°F+
No Pre-Wet	Weeks-Months	About 10 Days	About 6 Days
No Washdown			
No Pre-Wet	* (No Data)	About 5 Days	About 5 Days
15-Minute Washdown			
Pre-Wet and 15-Minute Washdown	Several Hours Or Less *	Several Hours	Several Hours

SOURCE: NSTM Chapter 470, 2006.

Table 3.7 H-Blister Agent: Time to Decontaminate Ships' Decks

Countermeasure Washdown (CMWD) Situation	Wind Across Deck Area (Knots)	Estimated Deck Temperature		
		30°F	60°F	90°F+
No Pre-Wet	0 to 4	72:00 +	24:00 +	6:00
No Washdown	5 to 20	20:00	4:00	1:00
	21 to 40	12:00	3:45	0:55
	Over 41	10:00	3:30	0:50
No Pre-Wet	0 to 4	18:00	2:00	1:45
15-Minute Washdown	5 to 20	2:45	1:15	0:30
	21 to 40	2:30	1:15	0:30
	Over 41	2:00	1:00	0:25
Pre-Wet and 15-Minute Washdown	0 to 4	9:00	1:15	0:30
	5 to 20	1:30	1:00	0:20

SOURCE: NSTM Chapter 470, 2006.

Table 3.8 G-Nerve Agents: Time to Decontaminate Ships' Decks

Countermeasure Washdown (CMWD) Situation	Wind Across Deck Area (Knots)	Estimated Deck Temperature		
		30°F	60°F	90°F+
No Pre-Wet	0 to 4	48:00 +	6:00	2:00
No Washdown	5 to 20	3:00	0:45	0:35
	21 to 40	2:30	0:40	0:30
	Over 41	2:00	0:35	0:25
No Pre-Wet	0 to 4	18:00	2:15	1:15
15-Minute Washdown	5 to 20	1:15	0:20	0:20
	21 to 40	1:15	0:20	0:20
	Over 41	1:00	0:20	0:20
Pre-Wet and 15-Minute Washdown	0 to 4	0:20	0:20	0:20
	5 to 20	0:20	0:20	0:20
	21 to 40	0:20	0:20	0:20
	Over 41	0:20	0:20	0:20

SOURCE: NSTM Chapter 470, 2006.

Summary

The Navy's capability to recover contaminated forces is currently limited by the rates included in Table 3.9.

Table 3.9 Throughput Rate to Recover Contaminated Forces

Activity	Platform	Rate (service members / hour)
Transport forces from shore to ship (Litter : ambulatory)	CH-46	26 : 39
	CH-53E	45 : 98
	LCAC: Passenger configured	100 : 200
	LCU	33 : 130
Decontaminate patients at sea base	LHD-1	12
	LPD-17	12
	LPD-4, LSD	0
Receive patients at medical department (total : surgical)	LHD-1	See RR-155/1
	LPD-17	
	LPD-4, LSD	N/A
Decontaminate ambulatory and uninjured personnel	LHD-1	60
	LPD-17	30

While no data exist to estimate the time required to decontaminate landing craft and aircraft, prospects to decontaminate these craft are known (Table 3.5). In general, landing craft are easier to decontaminate than aircraft.

When ships' CMWDS have been activated to pre-wet exterior surfaces, persistent hazards such as liquid chemical agents can be removed within several hours, and in some cases as quickly as 20 minutes.

4. Methods to Increase Navy Capability

Chapter 3 discussed the capacity of the Navy to transport and decontaminate amphibious forces at the sea base and the prospects to return ships and connectors to full mission capability. This chapter considers the order in which policy decisions guiding each of the activities should be made and methods the Navy can employ to increase its capability. The section is organized around policy options to address the following five concerns:

1. *Which amphibious assault ship should receive contaminated forces*? Each ship in the battle group has different decontamination and medical department capabilities, which must be well understood before recovery decisions are made.
2. *Which connector is best to go ashore and bring forces back to the sea base?* Air and sea craft may be contaminated while recovering ashore forces. Therefore, it is necessary to determine whether a landing craft air cushion (LCAC), landing craft utility (LCU), or aircraft (and which model of aircraft) can best withstand contamination as well as return the forces quickly and safely.
3. *What procedures should be used to decontaminate the forces when they arrive aboard the ships?* Forces should be decontaminated quickly so that their conditions do not worsen, and the spread of contaminants throughout the ship should be minimized. Decontamination procedures should be managed to maximize ships' ability to maintain and return to fully military capability.
4. *What is the prognosis for connectors and ships returning to full military capability in support of the mission?*
5. *Will the ships be required to return to port for reconstitution?* Or can ships remain at sea to continue the mission?

Which Amphibious Assault Ship Should Receive Contaminated Forces?

The ship selected to receive forces should have sufficient capacity in its medical department to receive patients in a reasonable amount of time. If there is sufficient manpower in the battle group to operate medical departments on multiple amphibious assault ships simultaneously, recovering forces to more than one ship should be considered to maximize medical departments' patient throughput. But this option is only available if each ship is manned with a fleet surgical team.

Using multiple ships, however, exposes more components of the battle group to contamination, which can divert those ships from their primary mission for a period of time if ship decontamination procedures must take place. Therefore, in order to minimize the opportunity cost to the battle group, forces should be recovered to one amphibious assault ship if possible, and to a ship that can receive casualties in a reasonable amount of time. How much time is reasonable is hard to predict in advance of an event; it must be determined by the battle group commander based on operational conditions. In general, it is suggested that an LHD be used to receive forces when more than five casualties require urgent medical attention.

Which Connector Is Best to Go Ashore and Bring Forces Back to the Sea Base?

Throughput and Speed

Table 3.1 lists the capability of each of the connectors included in the study, based on the number of passengers each connector can transport from shore to ship—including time to load and unload passengers. Considering the size and type of affected populations in this study, the time to recover contaminated ashore forces is displayed in Figure 4.1. (Assumptions made in these calculations are listed following Table 3.1.)

Figure 4.1 Time for Connectors to Recover Forces

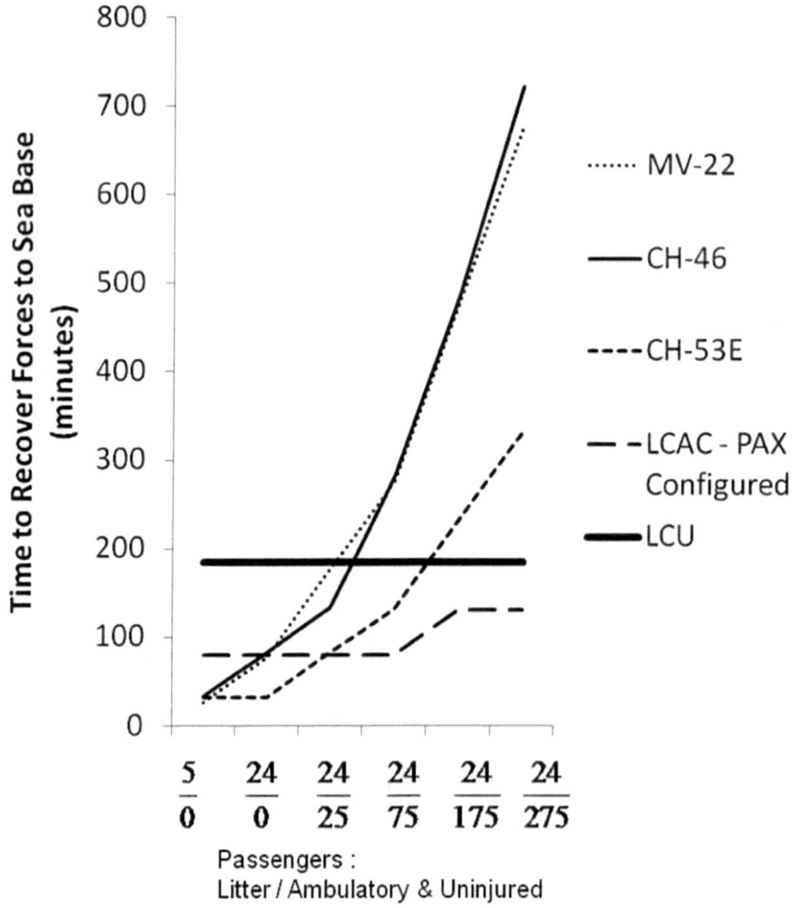

The minimum time to recover forces is achieved using aircraft, CH-46, CH-53E, and MV-22. Each of these aircraft can fly one sortie to recover forces in approximately 30 minutes. The landing craft included in the study, LCAC and LCU, at a minimum require approximately 70 minutes and 190 minutes, respectively, to perform one sortie to recover forces. In cases where there are casualties requiring urgent medical attention, the difference between 30 minutes spent in an aircraft and 70 or 190 minutes spent in a landing craft may affect the outcome of these casualties. It is recommended that aircraft be used to recover forces when there are casualties who require urgent medical care (Table 4.1).

Table 4.1 Recommended Connectors

Number of Passengers (Litter : Ambulatory)	Connector
Less than 15 : 22	CH-46
Less than 24 : 52	CH-53E
Less than 110 : 220	LCAC, passenger config. CH-46 or CH-53E for urgent casualties
Greater than 110 : 220	LCU CH-46 or CH-53E for urgent casualties

When the number of contaminated forces to recover exceeds the passenger capacity of a single craft performing a single sortie, it is recommended that the next-largest-capacity connector be used. This policy will generally enable all forces to leave the shore as quickly as possible in a single sortie, and will minimize contamination to craft. However, operational factors may support using multiple sorties or multiple craft.

If there are casualties requiring urgent medical care and the number of forces to recover exceeds aircraft capacity, an aircraft is recommended to recover casualties and a landing craft to recover the balance of forces. As described in Table 4.1, when the number of passengers to be recovered exceeds CH-53E capacity, use of an aircraft and an LCAC is recommended. When the number of passengers exceeds LCAC capacity, an LCU should be used.[24]

[24] As with all actions to recover contaminated ashore forces, selecting a connector involves a risk assessment by the battle group commander. Using an aircraft to recover casualties requiring urgent medical treatment can be faster than using a landing craft. However, it is possible that a battle group commander may prioritize other missions requiring aircraft and use of the flight deck over the mission to recover contaminated forces, and select to recover all contaminated forces using an LCAC.

Opportunity to Decontaminate Forces En Route

There is no current process to decontaminate forces en route from shore to ship. In the course of interviews and literature review, a list of candidate options for decontaminating forces en route to the sea base was developed (see Table 4.2).

Table 4.2 Options to Decontaminate Forces En Route

Options	Pro	Con
No en-route decontamination	None	Maximizes burden and risk to ship
Remove gear on connector upon exiting	Contaminated garments remain on connector; reduces cross-contamination to sea base	Slows cycle time
Operational decontamination: JSLIST gear change	Return to fight dirty without affecting sea base	Does not eliminate need for full decontamination
Corpsmen perform operational patient decontamination aboard LCAC	May improve patient outcomes	Unknown efficacy to decontaminate; Unknown risk or benefit to patients
Reactive Self Decon. Lotion (RSDL) for gross decontamination	Reduces cross-contamination risk	Not tested for this purpose, degrades fabric, obscures masks
Full decontamination en-route	Mitigates cross-contamination risk	Insufficient room

Removing gear while on the connector is fairly simple. While en route, it may be possible for contaminated forces to perform steps 1 and 2 of the personnel decontamination process listed in NSTM Chapter 470. These steps are (1) Remove outer gear (such as load-bearing equipment, mask carrier, helmet) and perform gross decontamination of masks, boots, and gloves. Gross decontamination of outer gear is performed with M291 kits, or a calcium hypochlorite solution. (2) Remove over garments (such as jacket and trousers).

Gross decontamination of outer gear is generally recommended so that the gear may be used again and the spread of contaminants is limited. Forces may consider discarding contaminated outer-gear rather than decontaminating it in recovery scenarios. In scenarios where there is a risk to service member well-being, it is permissible to discard contaminated waste into the sea.

If forces perform these two steps while traveling on the connector, forces can proceed to the next steps in the process when the connector arrives at the sea base: (3) Remove inner garments and (4) prepare to shower. The option offers the potential benefit of reduced cross-contamination because forces can shed their contaminated outer garments rather than transfer them to the receiving amphibious assault ship. The option poses little negative implication other than forces potentially exiting connectors more slowly if going through final stages of removing outer gear.

Aboard an LCAC, a PTM can provide an area up to 40 feet long where passengers can ride safely on the craft's deck. This area is not large enough to create a vapor hazard buffer, so if inhalation hazards are present, service members will need to continue to wear their masks. However, it may be possible to receive casualties on the aft section of the craft and stage operational patient decontamination there, so that recovered forces can be decontaminated and progress toward a clean area in the forward section of the craft. Medical department staff, such as corpsmen, may be able to perform or oversee decontamination of the wounds of injured service members more thoroughly than can the service members themselves or their buddies. This may prevent further injury, and may allow changing JSLIST gear or placing casualties in chemical protective patient wraps. It may also permit greater opportunity to render care for conventional injuries once the risk of CBR contamination is mitigated. This process has not been tested, and it would need to be evaluated through exercises to assess its effectiveness.

Operational decontamination consists of forces removing contaminated JSLIST gear and putting on uncontaminated JSLIST gear. This process could be performed on connectors if space permits. While there are no recommended procedures for performing operational decontamination en route, the procedure for performing JSLIST gear exchanges is well defined in NTTP 3-11.26 for land-based forces. NTTP 3-11.6 describes methods to perform operational decontamination for personnel, including cases where the activity is to be performed by forces individually, with one or two buddies, or as a unit activity. Each of these methods has space and time requirements; based on operational factors, it is possible that they may be performed aboard an LCU. Should space and time permit and if clean sets of JSLIST gear are available, performing operational decontamination of forces aboard connectors can allow forces to return to duty without traveling back to the sea base and bringing contaminants back to the battle group. However, this option does not eliminate the need for forces to be fully decontaminated upon their eventual return to the sea base, and the connectors used in the operation will become contaminated.

Reactive Self-Decontamination Lotion (RSDL) has been proposed for use in gross decontamination. RSDL would be sprayed over forces, head to toe, to neutralize contaminants that may have settled on their protective ensembles. RSDL could be sprayed over forces as they leave the shore and board connectors to return to the sea base. Like HTH solutions, RSDL is known to require a short time to effectively neutralize chemical and biological agents. But sufficient time should pass while forces are en route to allow the lotion to have its effect. If this process were effective, forces could disembark connectors and board amphibious assault ships with a decreased risk of bringing contaminants aboard.

However, this procedure presents risks. RSDL has not been tested as a gross decontaminant. It has been shown to neutralize contaminants in local application but not as a spray to cover entire outer garments. RSDL is known to degrade fabric, which may cause protective ensembles to fail if it is applied broadly. Additionally, RSDL is very expensive, and it may prove to be prohibitively costly to adopt this process as a recommended concept of operations and equip all Navy ships with sufficient materiel.

Lastly, performing full personnel decontamination en route may present a great opportunity to mitigate the risk of cross-contamination from recovered forces to the sea base. However, full personnel decontamination typically involves showers or wash stations and requires sufficient space to create a hazard buffer where decontaminated personnel may gather upwind of remaining threats. It is unlikely that sufficient space would be available on the connector selected for the mission.

The studied procedures for implementing decontamination processes aboard connectors did not reveal great opportunities to increase capability by reducing the risk of bringing contaminants aboard receiving ships. However, shedding contaminated outer garments before boarding amphibious assault ships presents a moderate gain in capability by decreasing the risk of cross-contamination. If sufficient space is available, removing outer garments appears to be a feasible option, and should be considered. Navy medical staff may direct corpsmen to perform designed patient decontamination procedures while en-route from shore to ship enabling greater opportunities to care for conventional injuries. Additionally, the use of RSDL for gross decontamination is a potential for further study.

What Procedures Should Be Used to Decontaminate the Forces When They Arrive Aboard the Ships?

Developing capability to increase throughput to decontaminate forces represents the greatest opportunity for the Navy to increase its capability to recover contaminated forces. Currently, there are no new decontamination technologies for the Navy to adopt.

RAND recommends that the Navy increase its ability to decontaminate litter patients by staging expedient deck decontamination stations. Doing so increases the throughput rate for patient decontamination and keeps contaminants toward the downwind aft section of amphibious assault ships, expediting the process to decontaminate ships and return them to full military capability. This process also keeps liquid and vapor hazards away from fore sections of the ship so that a vapor hazard buffer may be established, and flight crews and other ship's crew may operate without JSLIST gear.

Patient Decontamination Stations

Both large-deck and small-deck amphibious assault ships possess only one patient decontamination station, which can process twelve service members per hour. In the scenarios where 24 litter patients are recovered, it would take two hours to decontaminate all patients using the existing patient decontamination stations.

While an uninjured service member can remain safely in JSLIST gear for hours without sustaining any further injury from contaminants that may be present, service members who have suffered traumatic injuries will have damaged gear that is no longer fully effective at preventing further injury from CBR hazards. Urgent patients may have better outcomes if they are able to more quickly remove JSLIST gear and proceed to decontamination, thus freeing them from further contact with hazardous agents.

Additionally, once JSLIST gear is removed, injured patients can be more easily monitored, ensuring that they remain stable while awaiting higher-level medical treatment. Patients' status may change, and they may need to be re-triaged if their conditions worsen. Medical staff such as hospital corpsmen will be better able to monitor patients for triage if patients are out of their JSLIST gear. For these reasons, it is recommended that Navy ships stage expedient deck patient decontamination stations to increase decontamination throughput.

Staff on amphibious assault ships should construct expedient deck patient decontamination stations that employ the same procedures as the patient decontamination stations already present. Using simple tables, ships' crew can construct a three-stage process in which litter bearers or other crew cut patients out of their protective gear and decontaminate patients while medical department representatives inspect patients to ensure that they are decontaminated.

If conditions permit, staging these expedient deck patient decontamination stations on the aft of the flight deck, in close proximity to where casualties have been recovered by aircraft is preferred. On the aft section of the flight deck, liquid hazards carried with contaminated forces will remain on the surface of the flight deck and can easily be washed with the CMWDS after patients have been decontaminated and the aft flight deck is cleared.

Keeping contaminants aft of the superstructure on LHDs will allow continued operations on the fore sections of the ship, including flight operations. As such, flight operations can continue without requiring service members to wear JSLIST gear. Additionally, if no hazards are detected, crew may enter and exit the interior of the ship without using decontamination stations. Figure 4.2 illustrates the proximity of these activities on an LHD flight deck.

Figure 4.2 Expeditionary Patient Decontamination Stations on a LHD

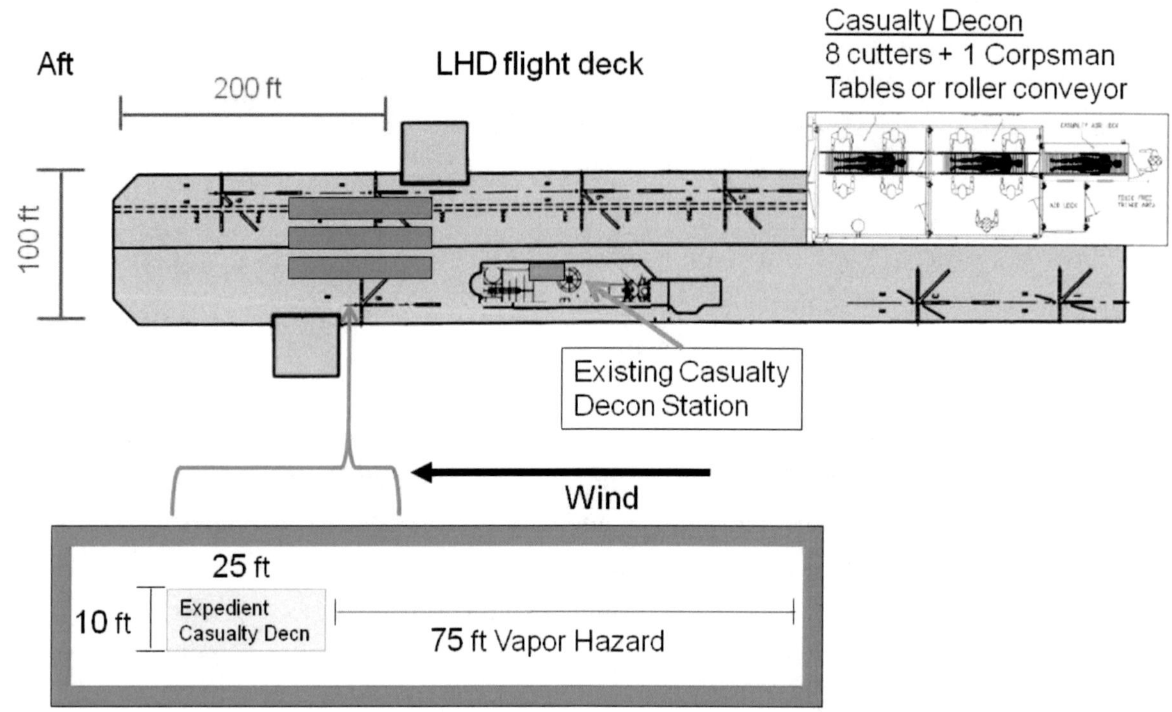

The upper right corner of Figure 4.2 depicts the process to perform patient decontamination in the existing patient decontamination stations on amphibious assault ships. The process performed in the permanent patient decontamination stations involves eight litter bearers to cut the patient out of his or her outer garments and decontaminate the individual while a representative from the damage control team supervises. In the third stage, a representative from the medical department checks to ensure that the patient is decontaminated. The patient decontamination area can be set up in a space approximately 10 feet by 25 feet. Given those dimensions, three expedient decontamination stations can be set up on the aft section of the flight deck. It is recommended that three stations be constructed so that 24 contaminated litter-bound patients can be decontaminated in under an hour.

Figure 4.2 also shows that expedient patient decontamination stations should be kept 75 feet downwind of other forces to maintain a vapor control area.[25] In current Navy guidance for performing decontamination aboard ship, there is no instruction that locating decontamination areas on the aft section of a flight deck (or near the stern gate in a well deck) can prevent a vapor hazard from reaching other areas of the ship. If sensors are placed upwind from the vapor hazard, and confirm that no vapor hazard is present, ships' crew should be able to operate outside the CPS without JSLIST gear. This would greatly

[25] Army SBCCOM, 2000.

increase their ability to perform their duties; they could work for longer than would be feasible given work/rest cycles for forces wearing JSLIST gear. Service members would be able to enter and exit fore areas of the ship that are secluded in the CPS without going through decontamination stations.

The same process can be implemented if contaminated patients are recovered to a small-deck amphibious assault ship, such as a LPD-17. Staging expedient patient decontamination stations on the flight deck will expedite urgent casualty decontamination and allow ships' CMWDS to easily decontaminate when the process is completed. The flight deck on a LPD-17 is approximately 200 feet and includes a fore and aft aircraft landing position. Navy damage control and flight deck crew should exercise options to land an aircraft with contaminated forces and establish expedient patient decontamination stations to see if sufficient space (approximately 75 feet) is available with the aircraft in either the fore or aft position, to create a sufficient buffer to present vapor hazards from reaching other areas of the ship.

If conditions threaten staging expeditionary decontamination stations on the flight deck, the Navy should consider the following options, in order.

1. Create temporary shelters to allow patient decontamination operations on the flight deck (include heaters if climate control is necessary).
2. Locate expeditionary patient decontamination stations on the leeward catwalk where they are sheltered from the weather; the area can be easily decontaminated using the CMWDS after the process is finished.
3. Stage expeditionary patient decontamination stations in the hangar deck, near the elevator. There, urgent casualties can be decontaminated quickly, but decontaminating the area will be more challenging.

Personnel Decontamination

Damage control staff are currently trained to perform personnel decontamination by setting up a CCA in close proximity to where forces enter the ship. After removing recovered forces' outer gear and outer garments, damage control crew escort them along a marked path toward the existing personnel decontamination stations and use the stations to process the contaminated forces. For populations of recovered forces, such as the several hundred service members included in the scenarios for this study, current procedures would require hours to complete personnel decontamination. During this process, damage control crew members would recommend that the entire ship's crew remain in the CPS or wear JSLIST gear.

By establishing expedient showers near the area where forces board an amphibious assault ship, the Navy can gain capability by keeping liquid and vapor contaminants from permeating throughout the ship and can perform personnel decontamination much more quickly.

In the case where ambulatory and uninjured forces arrive on the aft section of the flight deck, fire hoses outfitted with fog nozzles that reduce pressure to around 60 pounds per square inch can be used as showers. Showers should be directed so contaminated runoff drains off the ship. After service members finish showering, they can walk upwind toward the fore section of the flight deck and the superstructure into an area free of any hazards. With this procedure, all liquid and vapor hazards remain on the aft section of the flight deck and do not interrupt operations in other areas of the ship.

In the case where forces are recovered and arrive via landing craft in the well deck, damage control crew can stage expedient showers using either the well deck sprinkler systems or fire hoses and fog nozzles to create mass showers, as recommended for civilian emergency response in Army Soldier and Biological Chemical Command (SBCCOM) Guidelines.

If wind generated through the well deck exits out the aft section of the ship, the area forward of the well deck is beyond the vapor hazard area. This area includes the lower vehicle area and the balance of the ship. Medical department personnel should meet recovered forces beyond the vapor hazard area to monitor their health and ensure that they are free of contaminants. Here, the ship's crew can work free of protective gear, including gas masks, as long as there is no detectable vapor hazard present.

The SBCCOM Guidelines recommend that approximately 100 persons per hour can process through an expedient shower area ten feet in width. By extension, a shower area three times that width, which is established in the well deck of an amphibious assault ship, can be conservatively estimated to process 300 service members in an hour.

Figure 4.3 Increase in Decontamination Throughput with Expedient Deck Patient Decontamination Stations and Decontamination Showers

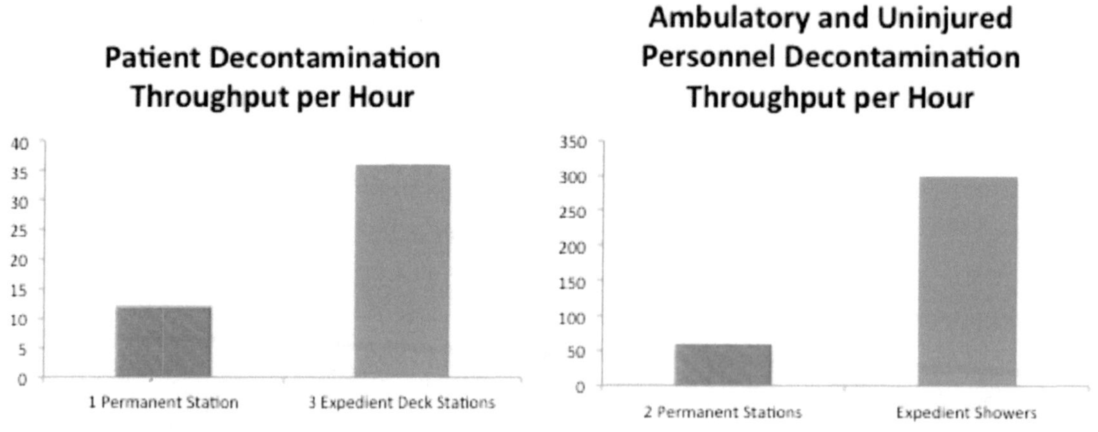

What Is the Prognosis for Connectors and Ships Returning to Full Military Capability in Support of the Mission?

If contaminated patients are brought to existing patient decontamination stations, contaminants will be brought within the skin of the ship. Damage control crews have procedures to decontaminate interior spaces. It is a manual process that consists of scrubbing and swabbing contaminated areas with HTH solution. Ships' crew members must wait for the solution to neutralize contaminants. Following neutralization, the area is rinsed, the solution is safely disposed of, and the area is tested to ensure that it is no longer contaminated. This process does not have defined estimates for duration.

When litter-bound casualties are decontaminated in expedient deck patient decontamination stations staged on the flight deck, contaminants are kept out of interior spaces. Ships' crews can be assured that CMWDS will effectively remove contaminates as quickly as they can (Tables 3.6–3.8).

This study does not define any new capabilities to improve connector decontamination. (Table 3.5 lists the prospects to decontaminate connectors.) Landing craft can generally be decontaminated more easily than aircraft. Selecting landing craft to recover contaminated forces can ease connector decontamination.

Will the Ships Be Required to Return to Port for Reconstitution?

Using CMWDS to remove contaminants from ships' exterior surface and decontaminating interior spaces with HTH solution, ships' damage control crew can thoroughly decontaminate ships so that they can continue their mission without returning to port for decontamination.[26] When radiological contamination persists, military guidance recommends that service members may work free of JSLIST gear when readings are below 0.33 centigray per hour.[27] However, ships face a persistent threat of cross-contamination when recovered forces have been infected with biological agents. In order to remain at sea without returning to port to offload contagious passengers, ships must plan to isolate them from the uninfected crew.

Biological Hazard Isolation

The Navy has long been concerned with the lack of capability aboard ships to isolate contagious service members. The outcomes and conclusions of a Navy exercise involving shipboard patient isolation are described in RR-155/1.

---

[26] Crew members should be diligent in ensuring that hazards have been neutralized or removed. Residual contamination can create a persistent off-gassing or reaerosolization hazard.

[27] FM 3-5/MCWP 3-37.3, July 2000.

A military utility assessment in August 2010 stated a need for the Navy to define the requirement for shipboard isolation of contagious patients. Such isolation could be achieved by procuring commercially developed portable anterooms and/or pack-up kits that present a fully portable quarantine capability. The assessment concluded that Navy should proceed to develop this capability for all classes of Navy ships.[28]

The research team performed literature reviews and conducted interviews to gather data to assess quarantine aboard ship. The first step in this process was to define the mission, using clinical definitions of patient isolation. Biological hazards were categorized based on the type of isolation capability required to prevent cross-contamination: standard, contact, and airborne.[29] Table 4.3 lists examples of toxins that fall into each of these categories and gives a brief description of the isolation protocols necessary in each case.

Table 4.3 Biological Hazards Defined by Necessary Type of Precaution

Type of Precaution:	Standard	Contact	Airborne
Necessary Procedures:	Wash hands, mask, eye protection	Wear gloves for all patient contact	Negative pressure, HEPA filter
Examples:	Tularemia, Ricin	T-2 Mycotoxins, Bubonic Plague	TB, Smallpox

Biological hazards requiring standard and contact precautions can be easily isolated with the current medical department capabilities present aboard Navy amphibious assault ships. Standard and contact precautions can be implemented using protective garments already provided to ships' medical departments. The precautions necessary to prevent cross-contamination for hazards requiring airborne precautions pose a challenge for Navy ships.

When patients are infected with biological hazards such as smallpox, exhaled airborne toxins can infect unprotected service members. In order to safeguard against cross-contamination, persons coming into proximity with infected individuals must take all standard and contact precautions and must don a face mask with respirator to protect themselves from airborne toxins. To isolate contagious individuals and prevent spread to others, it is necessary to quarantine the infected individuals in an area with negative

---

[28] Commander U.S. Third Fleet, "Forwarding of the Shipboard Isolation and Quarantine Experiment Military Utility Assessment," 11 April 2011.

[29] Droplet precautions is another category used in clinical settings for certain hazards. This precaution requires only slightly different protective garments from the standard and contact precautions, and all necessary garments should currently be present in Navy ships' medical departments. So this category of protocols is not explicitly addressed.

pressure, and use High-Efficiency Particulate Air (HEPA) filters to purify air that may contain contaminants.

Table 4.4 lists several options to address these challenges, along with the strengths and risks of each. If deck space is available outside the CPS and downwind, locating contaminated service members in this area presents a very good option. It ensures that biological agents will not enter the CPS to infect other crew members and permits crew members to enter and exit the CPS through fore and upwind locations without using airlocks.

Table 4.4 Options to Prevent Airborne Biological Hazard Cross-Contamination

Policy Option	Pro	Con
Outfit crew with N95 respirators	No infrastructure changes necessary	Uncertain effectiveness of long-term respirator use; negative impact on crew effectiveness
Establish temporary shelters		
Berthing / Medical Department	Comfortable for patients, nearby to medical staff	Require anteroom for enter/exit – may require HEPA filters added for interior areas
Pop-up shelters, Outside CPS	Crew working nearby may not need respirators; may not need airlocks to enter/exit CPS	Capacity may be very small; require ships to carry dedicated materiel for this capability
Deck, outside CPS and downwind	Crew may be able to enter/exit CPS upwind without using airlocks	May use space necessary for vehicles and equipment; require crew in these areas to wear respirators
Focsle, outside CPS and upwind	Area may not be as mission critical as deck space	Upwind location, may require all crew outside CPS to wear respirators; use airlocks to enter/exit
Create permanent space in ship's structure	No crew respirators or airlock use required to enter/exit CPS	Expensive

5. Conclusions

The Navy's capability to recover contaminated and injured forces to the sea base during amphibious missions is limited by two primary factors. The first is lack of an efficient process to evaluate the operational environment and identify connectors and ships based on transportation requirements for the recovery operation. The second is limitations in the capacity and throughput to recover contaminated service members aboard ships.

Both of these factors have significant impact on mission effectiveness, as described in the previous sections of this report. The results of RAND's evaluation suggest that it is possible for the Navy to improve its capability by implementing the following recommendations:

1. Develop a decision process for recovery operations. Once it is determined that contaminated forces will be recovered to the sea base, the battle group commander must quickly decide which ship(s) will receive the contaminated forces and how they will be transported to the ship. A critical factor in the selection criteria for a ship (or ships) is sufficient medical department capacity to treat contaminated and injured personnel. The total number of contaminated forces will also weigh into this decision.

The second decision that needs to be made is the selection of a connector (or connectors) to recover the ashore forces. It is recommended that an aircraft be selected to recover casualties in urgent need of medical care, and a landing craft be selected to recover large numbers of forces.

In addition, the location of decontamination operations must be determined, with the primary goal being to reduce the spread of contaminants. On the flight deck, decontamination should be performed on the aft deck to reduce the risk to aircraft and aircrews on the fore flight deck. It is also important to avoid landing additional aircraft near decontamination operations to reduce the risk from rotor wash. Decontamination operations in the well deck should be performed in the aft well deck to avoid contaminant spread throughout the ship.

2. Employ expedient deck decontamination processes aboard amphibious assault ships to increase personnel decontamination throughput per hour. Set up expedient patient decontamination stations on the flight deck and expedient showers in the well deck. Such a configuration will speed decontamination, minimize the areas where JSLIST gear must be worn, and decrease the time required to thoroughly decontaminate and return the ship to full military capability.

The increase in throughput per hour is substantial using these recommended processes. Amphibious assault ships that currently have only one patient decontamination station could triple their capacity by staging three deck decontamination stations, so that they could process the greatest number of litter patients considered in study scenarios in 40 minutes. By staging expedient showers, LPD-17s with only one personnel decontamination station, and LHDs with two stations exiting into the CPS could reduce the time required to process 275 service members from nine and four and a half hours, respectively, to under one hour.

Implementing these recommendations will require some change in DOTMLPF. Primarily, the Navy needs to amend doctrine to strengthen guidance in these areas and train its forces to be familiar with and proficient at performing recovery operations. Minor changes are also needed to organization, materiel, and personnel. But overall, implementing these recommendations is well within the Navy's reach, as additional costs in terms of needed materiel and personnel are nominal.

In addition to these recommendations, the study identified potential opportunities for the Navy to increase capability when recovering contaminated forces in amphibious missions. First, develop and implement en-route decontamination procedures such as operational decontamination of patients, and use RSDL in gross decontamination. Second, use the capability provided by ships' CPS to isolate service members infected with biological agents requiring isolation or special airborne precautions, and create temporary shelters outside the CPS. All of these suggestions remain untested and unproven, and may offer the Navy enhanced capabilities if developed, tested, and proved to be effective.

The Navy has included operations to recover amphibious forces in CBR environments in recent tabletop exercises (Navy Craft CBRN Survivability tabletop exercise, August 2010), and in studies sponsored by RAND and CNA to address this mission. Isolating contagious service members has been studied at even greater length.[30] If the Navy incorporates such scenarios in its planning requirements, it could address its gaps in capability by implementing recommendations from this study.

---

30 Joint Requirements Office for CBRN Defense, *Shipboard Isolation and Quarantine Concept Experiment Final Report*, May 2011.

Appendix A. Navy Doctrine Relevant to CBRN Recovery Operations

The current doctrine relevant to the recovery of contaminated forces in amphibious missions includes the following:

Department of the Navy, *Naval Ships' Technical Manual Chapter 470: Shipboard BW/CW Defense and Countermeasures, Direction of Commander, Naval Sea Systems Command*, S9086-QH-STM-010, 2006b.

Department of the Navy, *Chemical Agent Casualties and Conventional Military Chemical Injuries*, FM 4-02.285/MCRP 4-11.1A/NTRP 4-02.22/AFTTP(I) 3-2.69, 2007.

Department of the Navy, *Multiservice Tactics, Techniques, and Procedures for Chemical, Biological, Radiological, and Nuclear Decontamination*, FM 3-11.5/MCWP 3-37.3/NTTP 3-11.26/AFTTP(I) 3-2.60 IX-13, 2006.

Department of the Navy, *Multiservice Tactics, Techniques, and Procedures for Installation CBRN Defense*, FM 3-11.34/MCWP 3-37.5/NTTP 3-11.23/AFTTP(I) 3-2.33, 2007.

Department of the Navy, *Chemical, Biological, Radiological, and Nuclear Defense NATOPS Manual*, NAVAIR 00-80T-121, 2008.

Department of the Navy, *Multiservice Tactics, Techniques, and Procedures for Health Service Support in a Chemical, Biological, Radiological, and Nuclear Environment*, FM 4-02.7/MCRP 4-1.1F/NTTP 4-02.7/AFTTP 3-42.3, 2009.

Department of the Navy, NTTP 3-02.1.1M, "Recovery Operations in a Chemical, Biological, Radiological, and Nuclear (CBRN) Environment," October 2011, Draft.

Appendix B. Doctrine Supporting CBRN Recovery Operations

This appendix contains specific revisions to Navy doctrine that would be required to implement the use of expedient deck decontamination stations, as outlined in Chapter 5 of this report. The recommended changes aim to clarify doctrine in the following areas:

- Decision process to recover contaminated forces in amphibious missions
- Method and location to perform personnel decontamination aboard amphibious assault ships
- Isolating contagious forces aboard ships.

Decision Process to Recover Contaminated Forces in Amphibious Missions

FM 4-02.7/MCRP 4-11.1F/NTTP 4-02.7/AFTTP 3-42.3; "MULTISERVICE TACTICS, TECHNIQUES, AND PROCEDURES FOR HEALTH SERVICE SUPPORT IN A CHEMICAL, BIOLOGICAL, RADIOLOGICAL, AND NUCLEAR ENVIRONMENT"; JULY 2009.

Chapter V, "PATIENT DECONTAMINATION"; 29. Establishing a Patient Decontamination Station on a Water Vessel. b. Shipboard Decontamination of Ground Force Personnel:

Current: This section states that ground forces should be decontaminated before they are transported back to a ship. In cases when they are transported dirty, they should be decontaminated on the deck of the receiving ship.

Proposed: This section should include the decision framework for recovering contaminated forces in amphibious missions.

Department of the Navy, Naval Ships' Technical Manual Chapter 470: Shipboard BW/CW Defense and Countermeasures, Direction of Commander, Naval Sea Systems Command, S9086-QH-STM-010, 2006b.

470-1.3.5 CONTROLLED INTRODUCTION OF CONTAMINATED PERSONNEL AND EQUIPMENT:

Current: NSTM Chapter 470 refers to NTTP 3-02.1.1 to provide instructions on recovery operations in CBR environments. At this time, the current version of NTTP 3-02.1.1M is in draft form only, not approved by any Navy command.

Proposed: NTTP 3-02.1.1M should be updated and approved for publication.

NTTP 3-02.1.1M Recovery Operations in a Chemical, Biological, Radiological, and Nuclear (CBRN) Environment, Edition October 2011, Draft.

This document is not currently approved by the Navy. Although a draft version, it is referred by NSTM Chapter 470 as the doctrinal reference for recovering contaminated forces.

2.7 DECIDING TO CONTAMINATE SHIPPING, 2.7.1 Principles:

Current: This section includes a decision framework that recommends recovering contaminated forces only if there are no options to decontaminate elsewhere.

Proposed: Add to the decision process criteria for selecting which ship should receive the contaminated forces, which connectors should transport contaminated forces, and what processes should be used to decontaminate forces at the sea base.

Method and Location to Perform Personnel Decontamination Aboard Amphibious Assault Ships

FM 4-02.7/MCRP 4-11.1F/NTTP 4-02.7/AFTTP 3-42.3; "MULTISERVICE TACTICS, TECHNIQUES, AND PROCEDURES FOR HEALTH SERVICE SUPPORT IN A CHEMICAL, BIOLOGICAL, RADIOLOGICAL, AND NUCLEAR ENVIRONMENT"; JULY 2009.

Chapter V, "PATIENT DECONTAMINATION," 29. Establishing a Patient Decontamination Station on a Water Vessel. d. Ship Ventilation Consideration:

Current: This section describes detailed procedures for avoiding contamination to ships' ventilation system. It is not clear which class of ship is referenced.

Proposed: Specificity to include procedures for all classes of amphibious assault ships is recommended.

32. Moving a Litter Patient Through a Patient Decontamination Station on a Water Vessel:

Current: These instructions should be consistent with patient decontamination procedures in NSTM Chapter 470, NTTP 3-11.26, and NAVAIR 00-80T-121 to avoid confusion. The document recommends that three patient decontamination stations be set up on the flight deck. However, the document states that the three deck decontamination stations should serve only to remove outer garments from patients prior to entering the three permanent patient decontamination stations for inner-garment removal and to wash off contaminants. Currently, there are not three patient decontamination stations on amphibious assault ships, only one.

Proposed: The document should be amended to include suggestions from Chapter 4 of this report, acknowledging that there is currently only one patient decontamination station per amphibious assault ship. The document also erroneously reports the number of conventional decontamination stations for uninjured personnel or ambulatory patients. The document states there are three such stations off the flight deck. Currently, there are only two such stations on a LHD, one on each of the starboard and port catwalks on the fore section of the ship.

33. Procedures to be Performed in First Compartment. d. Transfer the Patient to the Second Monitoring Compartment:

Current: This section states that a patient should remain in the purge compartment for ten minutes to remove airborne contaminants. This guidance differs from other sources. In NSTM Chapter 470, no minimum required time is stated. Also, damage control crew members assigned to amphibious assault ships and working with Navy surface warfare commands stated in interviews that only two to three minutes are required for a sufficient purge of airborne contaminants.

Proposed: Recommend consistency in guidance for the minimum time contaminated service members must remain in the purge section of permanent decontamination stations.

Staging personnel decontamination on the flight deck is the only process discussed for recovery operations in this document. The document should be amended to include a reference to NSTM Chapter 470 for a description of processes for performing ambulatory and uninjured personnel decontamination in the well deck.

Department of the Navy, Naval Ship's Technical Manual Chapter 470: Shipboard BW/CW Defense and Countermeasures, Direction of Commander, Naval Sea Systems Command, S9086-QH-STM-010, 2006b.

470-6.7.1.6 CPS Decontamination Station and CPS Casualty Decontamination Station:

Current: This section states that all personnel who are on a weather deck in a CBR environment must enter the CPS through a decontamination station.

Proposed: The document should be revised to state that recovered forces who are decontaminated in expedient deck decontamination station on the aft section of the flight deck, or in an expedient shower in the well deck, may progress to fore sections of the ship where there should be no vapor hazard. If recovered forces are checked by medical department personnel to make sure that they present no liquid hazard and have progressed forward of a vapor hazard control line into an area on the fore section of the flight deck where no vapor hazard exists, they should be allowed to enter into the CPS without going through a decontamination station. Enabling forces to move more quickly in and out of a ship's interior is a benefit of establishing expedient decontamination areas that limit the hazard presence to a confined area aboard the ship.

This doctrine should be amended to allow multiple types of threat areas, all outside the CPS. As in NTTP 3-11.23, a ship's commanding officer may designate upwind areas on the ship's deck to be free from liquid and vapor hazards. Reference *470-6.7.1.7 TP*

Zone Access in this document includes a table describing permissible methods to enter and exit a ship's protection zones in contaminated and uncontaminated environments.

470-7.7.5 SHIPBOARD DECONTAMINATION OF GROUND FORCE PERSONNEL. Refer to NTTP 3-02.1.1, Recovery Operations in a CBRN Environment:

Current: NSTM Chapter 470 refers to NTTP 3-02.1.1 for recovery operations. This document is currently in draft form.

Proposed: Reference should be updated when NTTP 3-02.1.1M is approved in final form.

CHAPTER 10, Decontamination, 10.8.1.2 Shipboard Aircrew Decontamination Procedures:

Current: Instructions for performing shipboard aircrew decontamination are consistent with decontamination procedures in NSTM Chapter 470 and NTTP 3-11.26.

Proposed: All three documents should be updated to recommend expedient deck decontamination stations and expedient showers, and should be made consistent with NTTP 4-02.7. Instructions in NAVAIR 00-80T-121 will continue to include detailed information for decontaminated service members wearing aircrew flight and JSLIST gear.

NTTP 3-02.1.1M "NTTP 3-02.1.1M Recovery Operations in a Chemical, Biological, Radiological, and Nuclear (CBRN) Environment, Edition October 2011, Draft"

3.3 CONTAINMENT PROCEDURES 3.3.1 Contamination Control Area:

3.3.4 Contamination Control Area Setup:

Current: These sections state that setting up CCAs in the well deck may require less manpower and materiel than in other areas of the ship such as the flight deck or hangar deck.

Proposed: Guidance should include recommendations so that in mass recovery missions, service members may discard over garments before entering the well deck.

4.4.3.1 Decontamination Showers:

Current: This section states that expedient showers may be necessary to serve large numbers of recovered forces.

Proposed: This guidance should be strengthened to include planning factors for circumstances under which expedient showers should be used: when contaminated forces are recovered from an ashore mission and it is possible to limit spread of contaminants to the area where recovered forces board the ship.

Fire hoses are recommended as a possible solution in NTTP 3-02.1.1M, but the document should list two primary options for establishing showers in the well deck of an amphibious assault ship: use fire hoses fitted with fog nozzles; and use the well deck sprinkler system, in the most aft position possible to allow a vapor hazard control area toward the fore section of the well deck.

CHAPTER 6, Naval Health Service Support Operations, 6.5 HEALTH CARE OPERATIONS:

Current: This section includes figures that display possible processes to decontaminate forces on the flight deck and in the well deck.

Proposed: This section should be supplemented with material from NTTP 4-02.7, which contains an authoritative discussion on patient decontamination.

The recommendation to establish expedient deck decontamination stations should be strengthened to make clear that patients may be fully decontaminated in expedient stations and moved to uncontaminated sections upwind of residual hazards.

Rather than recommend that personnel decontamination stations be staged in ships' well decks to decontaminate recovered forces, guidance should recommend expedient showers to quickly decontaminate recovered forces.

Isolation for Contagious Forces

Little guidance exists for establishing an isolation area for contagious service members aboard Navy ships. Isolation guidance should be added to NTTP 3-02.1.1M, NTTP 4-02.7, and NSTM Chapter 470.

Appendix C. DOTMLPF Implications

Implementing recommendations in this report has implications for DOTMLPF—doctrine, organization, training, materiel, leadership and education, personnel, and facilities—an overview of which is shown in Table C.1. This appendix describes the DOTMLPF implications in detail.

Table C.1 DOTMLPF Impact Overview

Area	Level of Impact	Description of Change
Doctrine	Major Impact	Define trade-off using connectors and ships for recovery vs. other combat activities; state process for expedient decontamination
Organization	Minor Impact	Shift personnel to augment medical department and conduct decontamination
Training	Moderate Impact	Establish and conduct training for expedient decontamination
Material	Minor Impact	PTM or MCESS, ladders, hoses, conveyors, isolation shelter
Leadership and Education	Unknown	Doctrinal changes and staffing will illuminate leadership impact
Personnel	Minor Impact	Adjustments to manpower throughout the ship/ESG in order to support simultaneous operations
Facilities	Unknown	Long-term effects on ships unknown; ships may need increased yard time for long term reconstitution

Doctrine

Changes in doctrine will be necessary to clarify processes and procedures if the Navy implements the decision framework and adopts the use of expedient deck decontamination stations and expedient decontamination showers. At least six documents containing relevant doctrine require modification. The aim of the suggested revisions is to clarify the following:

- The decision framework for recovering contaminated forces in amphibious missions.
- The criteria for selecting ships and connectors for receiving and transporting contaminated forces.

- Procedures to avoid contamination to ventilation systems for all classes of amphibious assault ships.
- Method and location for performing personnel decontamination aboard amphibious assault ships
- Revised procedures for performing shipboard aircrew decontamination
- Planning factors for circumstances under which expedient decontamination stations and expedient showers should be used
- Guidance for establishing an isolation area for contagious forces aboard ships.

Specific doctrine revisions are documented in detail in Appendix B.

Organization

Ships should organize the crew to have the correct manpower available to support personnel decontamination for up to 300 total contaminated forces, including 24 litter patients. Many of the crew members needed to staff decontamination stations are augmentees and need not come from any particular department. The manning requirements listed in NTTP 4-02.7 do include a specified number of medical department crew members. Staffing patient decontamination stations while receiving patients in ships' medical departments may require more medical department staff than are currently assigned to ships.

NTTP 4-02.7, chapter 5, section 30, includes a complete list of manpower required to set up a decontamination station (Table C.2). Using these manning guidelines, 13 medical department crew members and 41 other crew members are required to establish three expedient patient decontamination stations.

Table C.2 Patient Decontamination Station Manning

Job	Per Lane	For Three Lanes
Command and Control Cell		
Officer in charge.	1	1
Master-at-arms (May also serve as safety officer, or another individual can be designated. The master-at-arms also performs pat-down search and secures ordnance, and personal affects.)	1	1
On Deck Arrival Point		
Augmentees to remove litters (1 team of 4).	4	12
Primary triage officer (physician, PA, nurse, or senior corpsman).	1	1
Corpsman to administer treatment.	1	3
Augmentees to perform protective overgarment cut-off procedures. They wear TAP aprons.	2	6
First Compartment Decontamination Area		
Augmentees who cut off underclothing and decontaminate the patient. They wear TAP aprons.	4	12
Corpsman.	1	3
Second Compartment Contamination Check Area		
Augmentee trained to use various contamination check tools.	1	3
Corpsman.	1	3
Hot Line Patient Reception		
Augmentees to move litter patient out of second compartment across hot line.	2	6
Corpsman on clean side of hot line outside second compartment.	1	3
Total Medical	5	13
Total Augmentees, Others	15	41
Total Personnel For One Work Cycle	20	54

SOURCE: NTTP 4-02.7.

NSTM Chapter 470 lists work and rest cycles for service members manning decontamination stations (Table C.3). If temperatures approach 78 degrees F, the effective temperature for crew members wearing JSLIST gear will be 88 degrees F. Under these circumstances, a ship will effectively need twice as many crew members, working in 30 minutes shifts, to man decontamination stations. By these calculations, a ship will need to maintain 82 crew members who are trained to work at patient decontamination stations. Additionally, 26 medical department crew members would be needed to staff three patient decontamination stations with this work schedule.

Table C.3 Work and Rest Cycles for Crew Members Working in JSLIST Gear

Heat Category	WBGT [1], [2] Index (°F)	Light (Easy) Work		Moderate Work		Hard (Heavy) Work	
		Work/Rest [4], [5]	Water [3] Intake (Qt/hr)	Work/Rest [4], [5]	Water [3] Intake (Qt/hr)	Work/Rest	Water Intake (Qt/hr)
1	78-81.9	No limit	1/2	No limit	3/4	40/20 min	3/4
2 (Green)	82-84.9	No limit	1/2	50/10 min	3/4	30/30 min	1
3 (Yellow)	85-87.9	No limit	3/4	40/20 min	3/4	30/30 min	1
4 (Red)	88-89.9	No limit	3/4	30/30 min	3/4	20/40 min	1
5 (Black)	More than 90	50/10 min	1	20/40 min	1	10/50 min	1

1. Wearing all MOPP overgarments (MOPP - 4) adds 10° F to WBGT index.
2. If wearing body armor, add 5° F to WBGT in humid climates.
3. Hourly fluid intake should not exceed 1 1/4 quart, and daily fluid intake should not exceed 12 liters.
4. Rest means minimal physical activity (sitting or standing), accomplished in the shade if possible. The information pertains to acclimated service personnel.
5. The work/rest time and fluid replacement volumes will sustain performance and hydration for at least 4 hours of work in the specified heat category. Individual water needs will vary ±1/4 qt/hr.

SOURCE: NSTM Chapter 470.

Training

Interviews performed during this study included Navy staff responsible for managing CBR training with the following organizations: Surface Warfare Officer's School (SWOS) at Ft. Leonard Wood, amphibious assault ships, Afloat Training Group, and Assault Craft Unit. Training recommendations for each organization are outlined below.

Surface Warfare Officer's School

CBR instructors teach the Chemical Hazard Awareness Guide (C-HAG) course during SWOS. The curriculum includes lessons on the history of CBR weapons and the agents used, systems to detect agents, medical aspects, self aid and buddy aid, how to manage a ship's CPS, and CMWDS. Large group personnel decontamination is not covered in the curriculum. It is recommended that the C-HAG curriculum be expanded to include the capability to decontaminate populations that are large enough to stress the system, e.g., via expedient deck decontamination stations.

Amphibious Assault Ships

Navy staff interviewed for this study included damage control personnel, to include both officers and enlisted damage control assistants, and damage control petty officers. Consistent with NSTM Chapter 470, personnel described the ship's CBR Defense Bill as the guiding principles to which they trained, and by which they manage operations.

Damage control personnel currently train their crews to operate the CPS and the decontamination stations, run the CMWDS, and locate and eliminate local CBR hazards (essentially by laying down an HTH solution and swabbing it clean until no contaminant is detected). Current training does not support the recovery of large numbers of contaminated forces. It is recommended that additional training (in accordance with a modified CBR bill) be developed to practice setting up expedient deck decontamination stations for litter patients; setting up shelters on the flight deck or locating expedient deck decontamination stations in the hangar deck in case of inclement weather; recovering forces into the well deck as they shed outer garments and leave them aboard the landing craft; establishing expedient showers in the well deck using fire hoses or the existing sprinkler system; and using fog nozzles attached to fire hoses to stage expeditionary showers on the flight deck for ambulatory contaminated forces.

Also, additional ships' crew used in patient decontamination should train to perform these functions, to gain sufficient proficiency to decontaminate twelve patients per hour. Sufficient numbers of crew members should be trained in order to work in two shifts at three patient decontamination stations, as described in the Organization section of this appendix.

It is recommended that damage control staff organize training for flight deck and well deck crew, litter bearers, and other crew who are employed in ships' CBR response to practice the processes outlined in Chapter 4 of this report.

Afloat Training Group

Afloat Training Groups are stationed ashore and are responsible for training ships' crews between deployments. Afloat Training Groups should augment decontamination training to ships' damage control crews, so they may provide training similar to that for their crews with CBR responsibilities. CBR staff in the Landing Craft Unit (LCU) indicated they did not currently train with amphibious assault ships when in port. It is recommended that the Afloat Training Group organize consolidated training between the LCU and amphibious assault ships to practice transferring contaminated forces from landing craft to the well decks of amphibious assault ships while those forces are shedding contaminated outer garments.

Assault Craft Unit

Landing Craft Unit damage control staff also mentioned that they were familiar with performing CMWDS on LCUs. They are confident that the system will remove contaminants from the exterior of the craft, but they do not know the extent to which they will need to do additional decontamination to the interior of the craft or the best procedure(s) for doing so. It is recommended that LCU staff train the surface fleet to decontaminate landing craft with fire hoses, when the landing craft are positioned near the ships. This procedure is recommended in NSTM Chapter 470, and should be trained to be effective.

Materiel

The primary recommendations that require materiel development are in support of staging expedient deck decontamination stations on the flight deck and expedient showers in the well deck.

NSTM Chapter 470, section 7, includes a list of materiel required to equip decontamination stations aboard Navy ships (Table C.4). Additional respirators may be needed to prevent cross-contamination when isolating biological hazards.

Table C.4 Materiel to Support Decontamination of 100 Service Members

Item	Stock Number (NSN)	Unit of Issue	Conv. Station	CCA	CPS Station
Calcium Hypochlorite	6810-00-255-0471	6 oz.		48	48
Metal Trash Cans 32 gal	7240-00-160-0440	each	1	4	2
Plastic Bags 55 gal	8105-01-183-9764	100		25 bags	25 bags
2'x 2' X 6" Bootwash tray				1	1
Utility Pails (5 gal)	7240-01-094-4305	each		2	2
Pan, Steam Table (scissors)	7310-00-576-4614	each		1	1
Sponge, Cellular	7920-00-240-2555	each		3	3
Scissors, Bandage	6515-00-935-7138	dozen	2 ea.	10 ea.	12 ea.
Deck Brush, Scrub	7920-00-240-7171	each		3	3
Handle, Deck Brush	7920-00-141-5452	each		3	3
Boot Wash Brush	7920-00-255-7536	each		2	2
Gen. Purpose Detergent or Detergent Wetting Agent	7930-00-282-9699	gal	1	1	1
	6850-00-644-2008	50 lb	1	1	1
Measuring Cup (8oz)	7240-00-138-7983	box	1	1	1
M291 Kit	6850-01-276-1905	box	1	1	1
M8 Paper Booklets	6665-00-050-8529	each	4	4	4
M9 Paper	6665-01-226-5589	Roll	1		1
M256A1 Kit	6665-01-133-4964	each	2		2
Bench or Stool			1	1	1
Twine 1 lb. Ball	4020-00-231-5870	each			
Duct Tape, 2"	5640-00-103-2254	each		1	
Bags, Plastic 10 gal	8105-01-183-9765		100		100
Towels		each	100		100
Soap, bars			10		10
Hose Assembly, 3/4" ID	4720-00-230-6577	each			1
Nozzle, Hose Adjustable, 3/4"	4730-00-223-6731	each			1

SOURCE: NSTM Chapter 470.

Flight Deck

NTTP 4-02.7 includes a complete list of materiel required to set up a patient decontamination station in chapter V, section 31. NSTM Chapter 470, section seven, includes a complete list of materiel to supply decontamination stations. Materiel for expedient deck decontamination stations should be similar, with added materiel for tables and tarps to keep contaminants off the deck. In order to supply each of three expedient patient decontamination stations, three tables are needed, suitable to hold a litter patient.

Tarps in excess of 10 by 25 feet should be sufficient to serve as additional protection against contaminants pooling on the deck surface.

If expedient deck decontamination stations are to be set up in inclement weather, materiel for shelters should be provided. Shelters may be made of material already in place on ships, such as PVC piping and tarps. Space heaters should be available in case of cold temperatures.

The research team was not able to test procedures for assembling expedient patient decontamination stations. The Navy should exercise this process to fully develop the materiel requirements.

Well Deck

To establish expedient showers in the well deck using the existing sprinkler system, little additional materiel is required. To use fire hoses as expedient showers, the Navy should provide fog nozzles capable of reducing pressure an appropriate level for showering, around 60 pounds per square inch. Army SBCCOM (2000) illustrates how a corridor of expedient showers can be constructed with three ladders and two fire hoses with fog nozzles. If using fire hoses to establish expedient showers, the Navy should prepare to stage three such corridors in ships' well decks. In either case, garments should be provided for service members when they exit the shower area.

Damage control crew members were concerned that the wood planks lining some amphibious assault ship well decks may cause a persistent cross-contamination hazard if CBR recovery operations are performed in the well deck. Materiel should be developed to line well decks that can be thoroughly decontaminated by flushing with sea water.

Leadership and Education

There are no leadership and education recommendations at this time. As the capabilities are developed further, leadership and education implications may need development.

Personnel

Changes in ships' organizations to support operations to recover large numbers of contaminated forces in amphibious missions may alter the balance of personnel required aboard Navy ships. To the extent that these changes require a different balance of career fields, personnel management will be affected.

As in the Organization section, the majority of manpower required to staff patient decontamination stations need not be drawn from any particular department. Medical department staff members are an exception. Staff decontamination stations while receiving patients in ships' medical departments will place sizable demands on these staff members, and may require more of these staff than are currently assigned to ships. If more medical department staff members are assigned to ships, total Navy requirements for these manpower positions may increase.

Facilities

There are no known facilities recommendations at this time.

References

Department of the Navy, *Contingency Fact Book*, Washington D.C., Bureau of Medicine and Surgery, 2006a.

———, *Naval Ships' Technical Manual Chapter 470: Shipboard BW/CW Defense and Countermeasures*, Direction of Commander, Naval Sea Systems Command, S9086-QH-STM-010, November 1, 2006b. ———, *Chemical Agent Casualties and Conventional Military Chemical Injuries*, FM 4-02.285/MCRP 4-11.1A/NTRP 4-02.22/AFTTP(I) 3-2.69, 2007.

———, *Chemical, Biological, Radiological, and Nuclear Defense NATOPS Manual*, NAVAIR 00-80T-121, October 15, 2008.

———, *Multiservice Tactics, Techniques, and Procedures for Chemical, Biological, Radiological, and Nuclear Decontamination*, FM 3-11.5/MCWP 3-37.3/NTTP 3-11.26/AFTTP(I) 3-2.60 IX-13, 2006.

———, *Multiservice Tactics, Techniques, and Procedures for Health Service Support in a Chemical, Biological, Radiological, and Nuclear Environment*, FM 4-02.7/MCRP 4-1.1F/NTTP 4-02.7/AFTTP 3-42.3, 2009.

———, *Multiservice Tactics, Techniques, and Procedures for Installation CBRN Defense*, FM 3-11.34/MCWP 3-37.5/NTTP 3-11.23/AFTTP(I) 3-2.33, 2007.

———, *Chemical, Biological, Radiological, and Nuclear Defense NATOPS Manual*, NAVAIR 00-80T-121, 2008.

———, *Recovery Operations in a Chemical, Biological, Radiological, and Nuclear (CBRN) Environment*, NTTP 3-02.1.1M, October 2011, Draft.

———, Commander, U.S. Third Fleet, "Forwarding of the Shipboard Isolation and Quarantine Experiment Military Utility Assessment," to Commander, U.S. Fleet Forces Command (N9) and Commander, U.S. Pacific Fleet (N8), San Diego, April 11, 2011.

———, Office of the Chief of Naval Operations, *Required Operational Capabilities (ROC) and Projected Operational Environment (POE) for LHD 1 (Wasp) Class Amphibious Assault Ships*, OPNAV Instruction 3501.310B, June 2005. , Not available to the general public.

———, Office of the Chief of Naval Operations, *Required Operational Capabilities (ROC) and Projected Operational Environment (POE) for LPD 17 (San Antonio) Class Amphibious Transport Dock Ships*, OPNAV Instruction 3501.355, November 2005, not available to the general public.

———, Office of the Chief of Naval Operations, *Surface Ship Survivability*, NTTP 3-20.31/COMDTINST M3440.1, August 2011.

———, Office of the Chief of Naval Operations and Headquarters, U.S. Marine Corps, *Ship-to-Shore Movement*, NWP 3-02.1/MCWP 3-31.5, August 1993.

Joint Requirements Office for CBRN Defense, *Shipboard Isolation and Quarantine Concept Experiment Final Report*, May 2011, not available to the general public.

Los Angeles County Department of Public Health and the Emergency Medical Services Agency of the Los Angeles County Department of Health Services, *Terrorism Agent Information and Treatment Guidelines for Clinicians and Hospitals*, July 2006.

McGrady, Ed, "Resource Implications of CBR Use on Sea-Based Medical Casualty Management," Center for Naval Analyses, 2010.

Naval Surface Warfare Center Dahlgren Division (NSWCDD), *Navy Craft CBRN Survivability TTX Status Report*, May 2010.

U.S. Army Center for Health Promotion and Preventive Medicine, *Personal Protective Equipment Guide for Military Medical Treatment Facility Personnel Handling Casualties from Weapons of Mass Destruction and Terrorism Events*, TG 275, 2003.

U.S. Army Chemical School (USACMLS), *Multiservice Tactics, Techniques, and Procedures for Chemical, Biological, Radiological, and Nuclear Decontamination*, FM 3-11.5/MCWP 3-37.3/NTTP 3-11.26/AFTTP(I) 3-2.60, April 2006.

U.S. Army Chemical, Biological, Radiological and Nuclear School, and U.S. Army Edgewood Chemical Biological Center, *Guidelines for Mass Casualty Decontamination During a HAZMAT/Weapon of Mass Destruction Incident Volumes I and II*, ECBC-SP-024, April 2009.

U.S. Army Medical Department Center and School (USAMEDDC&S), *Multiservice Tactics, Techniques, and Procedures for Health Service Support in a Chemical, Biological, Radiological, and Nuclear Environment*, FM4-02.7/MCRP 4-11.1F/NTTP 4-02.7/AFTTP 3-42.3, July 2009.

U.S. Army Soldier and Biological Chemical Command (SBCCOM), *Guidelines for Mass Casualty Decontamination During a Terrorist Chemical Agent Incident*, ECBC-TR-125, January 2000.

U.S. Department of Health and Human Services, Radiation Studies Branch, Division of Environmental Hazards and Health Effects, National Center for Environmental Health, Centers for Disease Control and Prevention, *Population Monitoring in Radiation Emergencies: A Guide for State and Local Public Health Planners*, August 2007.